Your Mouth

A pragmatic exposé of informed self-care & astute
decision-making skills for the oral healthcare consumer

VE Adamu & NIF Eneojo

seasoned with some available current evidences about the
effects of oral healthcare interventions & researches

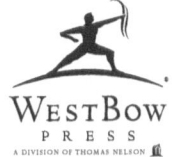

WESTBOW
PRESS
A DIVISION OF THOMAS NELSON

WestBow Press books may be ordered through booksellers or by contacting:

WestBow Press
A Division of Thomas Nelson
1663 Liberty Drive
Bloomington, IN 47403
www.westbowpress.com
1-(866) 928-1240

Scripture taken from the King James Version of the Bible.

ISBN: 978-1-4497-7826-2 (sc)

Library of Congress Control Number: 2012923497

Printed in the United States of America

WestBow Press rev. date: 01/07/2013

To our God, parents, siblings, children & friends

Table of Contents

Preface

A PALPABLE PERCENTAGE OF PEOPLE in our world are poor. Many of our communities are underdeveloped. To add to these, a lot of us are ignorant about matters that border on the health of the mouth. These factors have led to the increase we are experiencing in suffering due to problems of the mouth in the world today. Certain (relevant) national or regional health authorities have tried to reduce this suffering and improve quality of life for their people. However, their efforts, more often than not, have consisted of providing unplanned or scantily planned, ad hoc and spasmodic curative or educational services for the mouth's health, which in many cases are poorly distributed, and only rich, influential, or privileged persons or urban communities receive benefit from such care or program. Our authorities have good intentions; but we feel that they may not be using the proper approach to curbing mouth problems and reducing suffering for most people. On a general note, we have not been too committed to strategic long-term programs or efforts that foster better and livelier empowerment of the people to take reasonable responsibility for the health of their own mouth. If we are going to achieve what our authorities have failed to achieve, we must tackle our mouth problems from the individual/household level. We must empower people to take informed-responsibility for the health of their own mouth. Realising this need, we are placing this little book in your hands – and consequently, in your home - to help you understand your mouth better, prevent diseases of the mouth, deal with some minor ailments of the mouth at home and take good decisions when it is time to see people whose job it is to care for the mouth.

'Your Mouth' is a book written for everyone who has a mouth. This mouth-health information resource book is truth revealing and skills teaching. It is written from a rich background of years of experience in the delivery of functional healthcare to the mouth, teaching and research, and seasoned with some reliable research findings and evidences about the effects of care given to the mouth around the world. Our desire is that 'Your Mouth' would help you and your household to attain and maintain a level of health of the mouth, that will enable you to give full expression to the purpose of nature for giving you a mouth.

Current trends in healthcare delivery issues emphasize research, prevention and health care decisions based on evidences about the effects of healthcare interventions. It is our desire that you benefit from the advances in knowledge in these areas of healthcare delivery initiatives. The achievement of better health for the mouth requires the active, rather than passive, involvement of the receivers of care in the promotion of the health of their own mouth. Being well informed integrates you into this rewarding chore. It must be adventurous reading this book! Come on, and let us enjoy it, then!

- VE ADAMU & NIF ENEOJO
Enugu, Nigeria; October 2012.

1

Nature's Expectations

Nature does not change its course to sympathize with our ignorance or consequences of abuse. For instance, maize, rice, cowpea, meat, peanuts, etc. continue to need chewing before swallowing despite the fact that one's mouth is ailing. This means that nature does not expect us to lose our teeth or the tone and health of our gums, tongue, palate, cheeks and lips. She has given us a mouth. We must in turn do all we can to keep the mouth sound and healthy so it may serve us well.

THE MOUTH IS A REMARKABLE organ. It communicates many things that only actions can express. The mouth is a powerful tool for defense, assault, feeding, recreation, rehabilitation, expression, beauty, etc.

Several years ago, a colleague of one of these authors (VEA) was seeing a patient in a surgery opposite his inside a very busy mouth-care clinic in Owerri, one of Nigeria's eastern cities. She called his attention to a dilemma she was facing. She tried to convince a young patient who used tobacco to cease using it. Apart from the cosmetic concerns tobacco use posed to him, he stood the risk of losing the best quality of life he ought to live, later on, due to his potential predisposition to certain illnesses or even dying prematurely because of the health challenges tobacco use also confers on users. The young man forthrightly told her he had no plans to stay too long on earth. He wondered what he could be living for. He was ready to accept death any time it came, he said. This colleague of VEA was both confounded and stuck. She did not know what to tell him any longer. VEA also tried to convince the young man that he was courting a problem, all to no avail. She just had to let him be! Orientations can be that bad. You must value the gift of life to seek to preserve it. You must also value the gift of the mouth to seek to preserve it or benefit immensely from its use.

Just take a mirror (looking glass) and look at your teeth from 'molar to molar'. Do you like your set of teeth? What can you say about the colour and arrangement of your teeth? Now, look at your entire mouth. Note the teeth beautifully arranged on the two arches lining the corresponding jaws (upper and lower jaws). Immediately below the teeth in both arches are the gums. How do you like the colour of your gums? Can you see your palate? The palate is the roof of the mouth, overlooking the tongue, which, of course, is at the centre of the mouth. Can you also see the lining of your cheeks? We do not need to tell you that you have lips! All the structures we have identified above constitute the mouth.

Imagine, for a moment, a man without a mouth! Imagine how destitute of all mouth's potentials the man would be. You should feel the warmth of a deep-rooted heartfelt gratitude to nature right now - for having a mouth!

The mouth is a gift of nature - a natural resource. Nature has endowed us with many natural resources on earth. She has placed these natural resources at our disposal for our good. Think of the world without water or vegetation!

Grave consequences result from the abuse of any natural resource.

In many parts of the world, deforestation has contributed to desert encroachment. Many national governments are campaigning for tree planting activities geared toward reforestation. The use of forest trees for fuel is an abuse of the natural resource of the forest. What is the aftermath? Desert encroachment, soil erosion, etc. are all around us today as testimonials.

The abuse of the mouth, like any other natural resource, can have very serious repercussions. Diseases of the mouth such as tooth decay, gum disease, tooth loss, sores in the mouth, cancers of the mouth and mouth diseases associated with sexually transmitted diseases, HIV/AIDS and chronic diseases such as diabetes mellitus, etc. are major problems disturbing many people in the world today. A great number of these diseases spring from our abuse of the mouth. Many people are in pain and cannot really use their mouth the way they should because of problems in their mouth. This is saddening; but the most painful thing is that our carelessness and the habits of our lives cause most of the problems we have with our mouth.

Nature does not change its course to sympathize with our ignorance or consequences of abuse. For instance, maize, rice, cowpea, meat, peanuts, etc. continue to need chewing before swallowing despite the fact that one's mouth is ailing. This means that nature does not expect us to lose our teeth or the tone and health of our gums, tongue, palate, cheeks and lips. She has given us a mouth. We must in turn do all we can to keep the mouth sound and healthy so it may serve us well.

The mouth tells a lot about one's personality. A dirty, smelling or an ailing mouth introduces its owner as negligent, careless and uninformed. The cost of restoring health to the mouth and other possible crippling problems consequent upon lack of proper care should persuade anyone to care for his mouth. The entire mouth can be optimally functional for as long as one lives. If we are going to use our mouth as operationally as we ought to use it, a little more effort is required in our care of it.

Many mouths are ailing because:

- a lot of people have poor knowledge about the health of the mouth
- some people may be poor and are, consequently, not able to pay prescribed bills for the management of problems of the mouth
- many treatments for problems of the mouth involve a lot of 'time wasting' for 'busy executives'
- home-delivered services for the health of the mouth are rare or exorbitant
- people – at individual or household level, do not participate actively in issues that concern the health of their mouth and so they over-depend on people who are trained to care for the mouth.

Nevertheless, if we learn to (at home and at the household level):

- prevent diseases of the mouth
- recognize (dangerous) symptoms of serious problems of the mouth and seek treatment very early in their natural history; and
- promote the health of our mouth,

We will be able to:

- avoid many expensive attendances to mouth-care facilities or centres (clinics) ,
- cut down much time-wasting during routine attendances to mouth-care (dental) clinic

- care for our own mouth twenty-four (24) hours a day – and, at home! and
- preserve our mouth to serve us (optimally) for as long as we live.

2

Our Response

*Our response should be the resolve to avoid problems.
Avoiding problems should be the first level of care
we must give ourselves at home. Our goal should
be to promote the health of our mouth and to
improve aesthetics. Avoiding problems saves us
much pain, time, money and even embarrassment
that attend to some problems of the mouth.*

WHAT SHOULD BE OUR RESPONSE to nature's expectations? Our response should be the resolve to avoid problems. Avoiding problems should be the first level of care we must give ourselves at home. Our goal should be to promote the health of our mouth and to improve aesthetics. Avoiding problems saves us much pain, time, money and even embarrassment that attend to some problems of the mouth. Sometimes, it delivers us from reduction in quality of life or even premature death.

Think about the story of the man who set out to commit suicide by hanging himself on a tree trunk set in a nearby bush, who took to his heels as he chanced upon a python. You should wonder why a suicide-bound man would run away from one of the easiest routes out of this world, which he desperately wanted to exit. From the story, we can deduce that no normal, rational person really likes problems. No one likes the incapacitation of a toothache, for example. Everybody needs to attain and maintain a level of health that can stimulate productivity, creativity and ease in daily endeavours.

The health of the mouth is closely associated with the general health of the body. In fact, the health of the mouth is an integral part of general health and is essential to the overall health and well-being of all individuals. Have you ever noticed that when your body needs more water, like on a very hot day or when you work hard and are sweating profusely, you drink more fluid? Do you know that some elderly people, whose mouths are ailing, are malnourished or sickly or dying because they are not able to chew their food properly or even eat food or drink fluid because of pain and loss of tissue? What results? They are not able to get real energy or nutrients from food/fluid. A good look at the mouth could reveal symptoms of malnutrition, anaemia, infections, immune disorders, injuries, some cancers, etc. Caring adequately for your mouth could reduce your risks of some other general health problems. Recent studies have linked diseases of the heart, heart attacks, diabetes, fragility of the bone, HIV, adverse pregnancy outcomes, like pre-term pregnancies and under-weight babies, and strokes to diseases of the gum and supporting structures of the teeth, resulting from poor hygiene of the mouth. The early identification of diseases of the mouth may contribute to the early diagnosis and treatment for a number of diseases of the general body.

DAILY HYGIENE

One of these authors (VEA) remembers when he was much younger and in the primary (elementary) school; they had routine inspections of their teeth, nails, hairs, cloths, etc carried out by teachers on *assembly* grounds. Punishment awaited pupils who defaulted in a way or another. And so to avoid the punishment, pupils struggled to barb or comb their hairs very well, clean their teeth daily, cut their finger nails short, etc. It was a village school. If the teachers did not compel these pupils to observe these routines, the way they did, it is almost certain that many of the pupils enrolled in that school, then, would not have been diligent enough to comply with them. Even pupils who did not do these things normally, maybe, because of parental/guardian negligence or juvenile stubbornness/nonchalance, were forced to form these healthy habits because of the dire consequences of failing in any of the aforementioned disciplines. No doubt, some of the pupils were already practicing these activities at home; but even they had those tenets of healthy living consolidated as a result. Training and re-training of many of these pupils occurred, spontaneously, this way. You may be surprised to hear this!

It bemuses some of us who passed through such rigorous grooming when we see many adults neglect their activities of daily living – especially the cleaning of the mouth. You must learn and practice proper mouth cleaning regularly as we do most activities of daily living, in order to acquire the skills necessary for an effective job.

A clean mouth contains a host of bacteria (germs), and this number increases, many times over, when the mouth is not clean. Using saliva and fluid from the gums as their main nutrients, bacteria inhabit tooth surfaces, crevices of the gums, saliva, the tongue, and the lining of the mouth, threatening the health of the mouth, and even the body, generally. Mouth cleaning, therefore, is an important component of a healthy lifestyle.

The mouth requires daily cleaning. It is best to clean the mouth twice daily – last thing before going to bed at night and after breakfast in the morning. This practise effectively eliminates *dental plaque* and food particles from the mouth. Interestingly, this is one of the basic principles of preventing diseases of the mouth. Dental plaque is the sticky film of accretion, with abundant bacteria (germs) that constantly form on the teeth. This dental plaque is instrumental to the initiation of the two commonest diseases of the mouth known to man – tooth decay and diseases of the gum and supporting structures of the teeth.

Waking up in the morning, the mouth should be clean because of the previous night's cleaning. Operationally, the cleaning of the mouth should come only after having a breakfast. Rinsing the mouth with water before breakfast eliminates putrefying saliva and boosts confidence, though (Some people dread eating without cleaning in the morning!). If anything is eaten after this (morning's) cleaning, the mouth should be properly rinsed with water. In addition, one or two, or some pieces, of any of the fruits in season could be eaten after lunch as desserts, especially the fibrous ones, which some refer to as the self-cleansing fruits because of the belief that they help to clean the teeth as we eat them. The truth is that many of these fruits increase saliva flow to the mouth, apart from the mechanical cleaning possibilities they may whip up. The natural binding agent in the saliva, the *mucin*, could help bind up food particles from the teeth for swallowing. We are of the opinion that if fibrous fruits or desserts are any helpful in cleaning the mouth, they should be of little help. We advice, therefore, that regular cleaning and mouth rinsing should never be replaced with the munching of desserts – the so-called self-cleansing fruits.

Some persons have suggested cleaning the teeth after lunch. Some persons do practise it. Nevertheless, we have found no scientific evidence to proof that cleaning three (3) times a day is any helpful to the overall health of the mouth or harmful. The only thing we see in cleaning three times a day is that it may be hectic for people with very demanding schedules; it may not be cost-effective for some low-income earners and it may be unnecessary for the overall health of the mouth.

People in different cultures and at different times in history have employed various materials to clean the mouth. Some of these materials are: charcoal, cloth, sugar cane, fingers, river/sea sand, knives, sharp objects, nails, powder made from snail shells, bathing soap, gin or *'kai kai'*, mouth wash solutions, tooth picks, chewing sticks, toothbrush with tooth paste, etc, etc. All the cleaning materials listed here can cause varying degrees of damage to the mouth and they cannot clean the teeth properly, except the last two. Let us, at this point, take a methodical look at the two (good) cleaning materials.

Chewing Sticks

An African proverb says *'you don't use the chewing stick simply because you hate hunger'*! There is a specific purpose why chewing sticks exist at all. Chewing sticks are teeth-cleaning materials used in many developing parts of the world. They have been with man right from the beginning, obtainable fresh from trees and shrubs or bought at relatively cheap prices; the fresh or dry form may be used.

In continents like Africa and Asia, some cultural and traditional authorities believe that some chewing sticks have some medicinal properties. Some view certain chewing sticks as able to cure swollen gums; some others, mouth odour; still some others, general health problems. Experience has shown that some of these claims are true. For instance, using chewing sticks made from fresh 'bitter leaf' plant during and after certain illnesses remove coatings on the tongue – thereby improving taste; the plant acts as an appetizer to the convalescent patient.

A study conducted recently by one of these authors (NIFE) inferred that liquid and alcohol crude extracts of herbs known botanically as *Zanthozyluium macrophylla* and *Corchorus olitonius* showed antimicrobial activity against some *germs (streptococci species)* isolated from carious lesions (decayed teeth). According to this researcher, the overall finding of this study corroborates the use of herbs for medicinal purposes by herbal healers. That is, especially in dental practice! Similarly, another study conducted by researchers at the Osaka University School of Dentistry in Japan confirmed in 2008 that specific components of the essential oil extracts of *eucalyptus* are effective against *periodontal pathogens* (germs related to the gum and the supporting structures of the teeth). This research gives credence to the strong correlation between eucalyptus-impregnated chewing gum and periodontal health. 'Periodontal' refers to the gums and other supporting structures of the teeth. We hope that, someday, further research into these, and numerous other claims, would offer a better understanding of these herbs. Extracts from some local African or Asian herbs around may, one day, revolutionize dental practise and alleviate human suffering emanating from the mouth – far more than it has.

It is noteworthy, however, that some chewing sticks stain the teeth and gums and can constitute local irritation to them, initiating certain gum problems. Users of chewing sticks are to make use of the ones that do not pose any form of danger to the teeth and their supporting structures – and by extension, the entire mouth. We do not recommend the use of chewing sticks, though, except for persons or households that cannot afford to buy toothbrush(es) and toothpaste(s) always. The reason we do not recommend the use of chewing sticks is that chewing sticks are unable to clean the spaces in-between the teeth properly most of the times; and this predisposes those un-cleaned surfaces to tooth decay and, sometimes, some gum or other mouth problems.

To use a chewing stick, chew it to a consistency of tuft that would not injure the gums or harm the teeth or the entire mouth. Then, clean your teeth one after the other. For each tooth, give between 5 and 8 strokes – from the gum lining to the cutting/chewing edge of the tooth you are cleaning (in a one-way traffic manner). Do this for every tooth in the mouth on both the outer and inner surfaces. Only the chewing surfaces of the teeth you may clean in a 'back-forth', 'back-forth' manner. After this, run the tuft of the chewing stick over the gums with firm, gentle strokes, horizontal to the teeth outlay. This is termed, *gum massage*. Gum massage stimulates healthy blood flow in the little blood vessels of the gum and helps to toughen the gums against disease. Lastly, scrub your tongue with the tuft of the chewing stick (in a one-way traffic manner) from the back to the tip of the tongue; and rinse your mouth and the tuft of the chewing stick with clean water.

Toothbrush And Toothpaste

These are the best-known, appreciated and effective cleaning materials available today in the market for use. Many of the manufacturers of these toothbrushes did not seek advice from people trained to know about the health of the mouth and cleaning materials before they began production. The result is that we now have a lot of junks and bad brushes finding their way into our markets in the name of toothbrushes. You should be careful to buy a toothbrush that can clean the teeth very well without leaving regrets behind.

There are manual and automated/electronic toothbrushes. We recommend electronic or automated toothbrushes for people who are so handicapped, incapacitated, or challenged that they cannot use the regular, manual toothbrush. If you are to use an electronic toothbrush, you will do well to follow the instructions of the manufacturer of the type you purchase.

A good (manual) toothbrush should have a handle, which can be grasped in the palm (adult: about 6 inches long; children: about 4 inches long); then, it should have a small reasonable head (about an inch long for adults; and about 2/3rd of an inch long for children). The toothbrush's bristles arrangement should show well-separated strands of bristles and should be of medium texture for adults and soft texture for children. The brushing surface should be flat and the head of the toothbrush should run (tapered) smoothly towards the tip of the head-end of the toothbrush. This description fits a toothbrush that can:

- massage (the gums) well without injuries
- penetrate in-between teeth to clean dental plaque and dislodge food particles
- clean the teeth surfaces very well
- get to the last tooth in the mouth for its proper cleaning

Your choice of a toothbrush is the first most important issue in cleaning the mouth. Let us talk, a little, about the choice of toothpaste. The essential thing in a toothpaste, a part from the other ingredients, which, clearly, every toothpaste-manufacturing company 'worth it salt' would 'naturally' formulate hers to generously reflect, is *fluoride*. Fluoride is a chemical substance that helps to fortify the teeth against indiscriminate tooth decay. When you lay hands on any toothpaste, check out if it contains this chemical substance. If it does, you may buy it for your use. However, because many types of toothpaste labelled by their manufacturers as 'fluoride-containing' have been found to be without fluoride, it is best to buy toothpaste endorsed by one's nation's dental board or the World Dental Federation (FDI). Researches and experiences have taught us that many types of toothpaste may not do some of the work their manufacturers declare they can do after all. In some parts of the world, many claims on toothpastes may be advertorial in the final analysis.

For pleasure, it is good to buy toothpaste with a taste, colour and flavour and/or consistency that appeal to one. It is also good to change toothpaste immediately one discovers symptoms of allergic reactions to a particular brand in oneself or a household member. Symptoms of allergy may include feeling like vomiting, vomiting, unusual salivation, desquamation of the lining of the mouth (especially, on the lips), after using a particular toothpaste.

Now, let us turn to the issue of the technique of tooth brushing. As in many cases of skills-acquisition requiring manual dexterity, if you miss the technique of tooth brushing, you miss its 'blessings'. In fact, it is better to brush once a day in the proper (effective) or correct way than to brush twice a day incorrectly! The three most popular incorrect ways to brush are:

- to brush horizontally across the teeth
- simply brushing up and down the teeth
- brushing the teeth in circular motions

'How then may one brush correctly?' you may ask. Here is how: Get the correct toothbrush. Place some toothpaste on it. Lay the toothpaste-bearing bristles of your toothbrush against your teeth (upper or lower) in one cheek (right or left), sweep from the gums onto the teeth surface. Sweep in such a way that the entire length of the bristles have a sustained firm but gentle contact with the gum preceding the teeth and the tips of the bristles only slide onto the teeth surfaces to penetrate in-between the teeth. Repeat this action about 5 to 8 times in a particular section of the teeth (let the strokes be gentle but firm here too). A good toothbrush should engage about 3 teeth at a time. Then move to another section of your teeth and repeat the same things you did for the previous section and on and on, until you are done with the entire teeth in your mouth. You should brush two surfaces of your teeth differently. These areas are:

- the inner surfaces of the front teeth (in the upper and lower jaws) and
- the chewing/grinding surfaces of the teeth at the back of your mouth

For the inner surfaces of the front teeth, you are to place your toothbrush vertical to the long-axis of the tooth you wish to brush and brush the tooth from the gum to the cutting-edge of the tooth in a 'one-way traffic' manner. You should give each tooth 5 to 8 strokes of brushing in both the upper and the lower jaws. For the chewing/grinding surfaces of the teeth at the back of your mouth, you may clean the chewing surfaces of the teeth in a 'back-forth', 'back-forth' manner (two-way traffic). The teeth may afterwards be given single strokes of the toothbrush again and the tongue scrubbed (in a one-way traffic manner) from the back to the tip of the tongue; and the mouth is rinsed with clean water.

We would like to add these few words about how to take care of your toothbrush. Many authorities and toothbrush-manufacturing companies recommend that you change your toothbrush every three months or after some months. We do not share this conviction. You should allow two factors to guide your decision about when to change your toothbrush. First, you may wish to have your toothbrush changed when the bristles are not as firm as they were when you bought it. Second, you should change your toothbrush once the bristles are splaying. In order to increase the lifespan of your toothbrush, you may buy and use two at a time – one in the morning and one at night. The colours of the toothbrush's handles should help you to distinguish between which one to use and when. A good example is using a red one in the morning and a blue at night. When you are done with your toothbrush at any time, you should leave the toothbrush up-turned in a cup, with the bristle-end upwards so it can have sufficient contact with air, which helps to destroy some germs on the bristles. The habit of putting a toothbrush back into its manufacturer's pack after use should be discouraged.

Dental Floss Silk

The *floss silk* is a thread-like piece of silk designed to remove *dental plaque* and food particles from in-between the teeth. If used daily, it can considerably reduce your chances of coming down with certain gum problems and decays in-between your teeth. Floss silks are, consequently, an essential adjunct to the toothbrush. Many dental companies produce floss silks so you are going to find many brands of the product in the market. Manufacturers of floss silks often configure the product to perform certain other accessory functions or appeal to some groups of people. Therefore, you are going to find things like *waxed* and *un-waxed* dental floss silks, and minted and un-flavoured dental floss silks. They all work well. Choice of the type to purchase and use rests solely on the user or the user, in collaboration with his mouth caregiver.

To use a dental floss silk, cut a considerable length of the product (say about 18 inches) out of the bulk. Wind its both ends around both mid-fingers of both hands and stabilize it between the fore-finger and the thumb of both hands. Then negotiate the silk through the *contact point* (the place where two teeth touch each other) onto the open space in-between the teeth. Bend it around one of teeth, sweep in a zigzag manner for a time, then turn to the other tooth, and do likewise. Move to another space and repeat the procedure. Continue this way until you have cleaned all the spaces in-between your teeth. Then, rinse your mouth.

Many floss silks come in 'ready to use' forms these days. In this form, the length of the silk may just be about an inch. The silk comes, fastened to a little, fanciful plastic handle. There are usually several in a single pack. They are very easy to use. With this form all you need to do is pick one, grasp the handle well, slide the silk at the working end of the floss silk in-between your teeth and proceed with your cleaning as described above. With this form, the use of toothpicks may become outdated.

Medicated Wood-Points

These are special wood-points manufactured to treat the triangle-shaped gums in-between the teeth. The use of wood-points is often necessary after a surgery on the gums to take care of an advanced form of gum disease or trauma/injury. If you ever need to use a wood-point, your caregiver will tell you so and teach you how you may use it.

Mouth Rinsing

You should Endeavour to rinse your mouth after meals or after taking sugary/sticky foods. This helps to keep food particles off the teeth. To accomplish mouth rinsing, get some water into your mouth and gargle your mouth with it. You may wish to spit out or swallow the product of the gargling. It is as simple as that.

Toothpicks

We do not recommend the use of toothpicks. This is because they can create retention areas around the gums that can initiate certain gum diseases. Nevertheless, you may use the toothpick in certain special circumstances only if you can use it without pressing it on your gum.

Mouthwashes/Rinses

Mouth-rinses are intervention-driven mouth remedies specifically formulated to intercept some problems of the mouth. They are not supposed to be a part of one's daily hygiene. This is because they subdue or destroy certain microorganisms (germs) in the mouth. Continual use of these products can weaken or depress the organism targeted, giving opportunity to a "rival" organism to thrive and colonize the mouth, causing problems. A good example of this scenario is the weakening or killing of bacteria in the mouth by an anti-bacterial agent in a mouthwash, granting opportunity to *fungi*, another kind of microorganism, to thrive and colonize the mouth – giving rise to an oral condition called *oral candidiasis (moniliasis)*. Ideally, people should use mouthwashes/oral rinses under prescription from persons trained to care for the mouth and discontinue its use after the problem is resolved. To date, the best mouthwash/oral rinse solution is the warm water-saline mouthwash solution. This is prepared by pouring a tea spoon-leveled table salt into a cup of warm water and stirring until it dissolves completely in the water. This solution is useful in combating certain gum problems and enhancing healing after the removal of a tooth or after a patient has had a surgery. Warm water-saline mouth gargling is often recommended after one has had a prophylactic treatment, especially for patients with gum problems.

DESENSITIZING AGENTS

Desensitizing agents are mouth-care solutions or pastes formulated to assuage hypersensitive tooth/teeth. If a tooth or some teeth are hypersensitive, the owner feels a shocking sensation on it/them while chewing or drinking or talking or singing or the mouth is open. It can be discomforting. To relieve hypersensitive tooth/teeth, apply a desensitizing agent to it/them. The patient should discontinue the use of the agent after the problem is resolved. Chances are that some people may like to continue to use the agent long after the sensitivity is gone. A very good example of a desensitizing agent prone to abuse by people is the paste, *sensodyne*. A patient once told one of these authors (VEA) that she liked the paste so much and that it was her regular toothpaste! In fact, she had a lot of the product in stock as at the time we discussed. A relative abroad had sent several to her! You can just imagine how she felt when VEA told her it was not proper for her to continue to use the paste. The problem with such chronic use is that basically, the paste desensitizes tooth/teeth by stimulating secondary *dentine* formation. The dentine of a tooth is the layer immediately beneath the *enamel*, the outer layer of a tooth. The dentine partly determines the colour of our teeth - by how sparse or compacted our teeth's dentine is. When you continue to use this product, the production of more and more dentine is stimulated and as the dentine becomes more compacted, the teeth will appear darker and darker progressively. Sad enough, these stains are permanent.

SELF-CLEANSING FRUITS

Over the years, mouth caregivers have recommended that people take fibrous fruits after meals. These fruits, they believe, binds together food particles on teeth for ingestion. In this way, you rid the teeth of these unwanted particles and that they mechanically clean the teeth, too. That is why they are called *self-cleansing* fruits. We believe that these claims need some researches for authentication. Our only advice is that this practise should not replace mouth rinsing after meals or daily hygiene.

ROUTINE PROFESSIONAL CARE

In a study one of these authors (VEA) carried out recently about the way people demand for preventive services in a dental practice in Nigeria, he gathered that most of the participants attended the clinic because they had pain or a problem of the mouth that would not go away. Patients did not just attend clinic routinely for check-ups and/or prevention. This ought not to be so. It is best to visit the mouth-care clinic twice a year (6-monthly) for disease screening to detect incipient disease(s) and give prompt and appropriate treatment for the disease or condition and for routine prophylactic treatment. Some *Cochrane* review authors recently inferred that after reviewing the best available data on the subject, there was not enough evidence to conclude, regarding the potential effects of altering the recall interval between dental check-ups, that it is any good or bad. However, we still recommend that adults and children pay visit to the mouth-care clinic every six months. Persons at greater risk for diseases of the mouth (like those who have diabetes, are pregnant, who use tobacco or alcohol, have gum diseases, have poor oral hygiene and certain medical conditions) should visit the clinic more than twice a year (say quarterly or every four months or as determined by their caregiver).

When you visit the clinic, first, people trained to care for the mouth will review your case (professionally) and they will examine or evaluate your mouth properly. During this evaluation, these caregivers identify problems early in their natural history and arrest them. Secondly, you get to enjoy your routine prophylaxis. This professional prophylaxis is primarily professional cleaning of the entire mouth. Application of certain drugs such as fluoride gel can also take place, depending on your need. During cleaning, your caregiver cleans your teeth and gums. Anyone who does this is professionally trained to clean all the teeth in your mouth, both above and underneath the gums with no or minimal injury to your gums. You should not anticipate pains during cleaning as you would experience little or none, depending on the condition of your mouth. There are varieties of professional cleaning materials available in the market today. These materials may be electronic and they may be manual. No matter the one your caregiver chooses to use, all you need to do is just relax and have your treatment. Actually, this cleaning, professionally called *scaling and polishing* is the best treatment your mouth can receive in a mouth-care clinic. This is because if observed as religiously as we have prescribed here, it helps to prevent the two most common diseases of the mouth known to man – tooth decay and gum disease.

We should, as well comment here that persons going for surgeries related to the mouth, or tooth removal or tooth filling or most other treatments in the mouth receive the scaling and polishing treatment prior to the procedure. The professional name for this procedure is *pre-operative* scaling and polishing.

Before and after a scaling and polishing procedure, a caregiver will give you a set of instructions designed to help you care for your own mouth at home. These instructions are often more adapted to the special needs of your mouth than the ones we are giving in this book. Please look forward to these instructions whenever you visit the clinic. Should your caregiver skip it or forget to give it, do remind him as you pay for both cleaning and those instructions each time you pay for a scaling and polishing procedure; or you ought to.

TREATMENT APPOINTMENT(S)

Dental treatments are sometimes in segments/phases. The schedule of a single dental treatment could run for days, weeks, or even months! A patient may need to go back to the clinic for further treatments within a week or two of the initial treatment. These are what we call *treatment* re-*call intervals*. These appointments must be adhered to in order to get the best from a treatment course. The treatment appointments are not just arbitrarily scheduled. They are set out deliberately and skillfully to give you the best. The schedule of some procedures allows time for healing of tissues and resolution of swelling before further treatments can begin. Others schedules allow adequate preparation before beginning treatment. There are many other reasons for treatment appointments. Whatever the case is, your caregiver reserves the right, by his experience, training and expertise to determine how it is best for you to visit the clinic before a treatment procedure is complete, if you are not on a hospital admission.

CARE OF DENTURES

A denture refers to an artificial tooth. Special members of the dental team trained to fabricate artificial teeth do so using a special type of material that resembles a real tooth in strength and appearance and resembles the gum tissue in appearance. There are removable and irremovable dentures. There are also partial (to replace some teeth in the mouth lost to disease or injury) and complete dentures (for those who have lost all teeth in their mouth either due to disease or injury).

It is important to keep all dentures clean all the time. If you use denture(s), you must endeavour to clean it (them) as often as you clean your teeth or at least, once a day, using a denture brush or a hard toothbrush and toothpaste or soap and water. A stained denture should be soaked in a bleaching agent mixed with water for some minutes before cleaning. If there are bands on your denture, you have to carry it to the clinic for professional cleaning. When using a partial denture for the first time, you should wear it for about a week before ever removing it. This is to allow you get accustomed to it. Thereafter, you should always remove it before going to bed. This is to pave way for a good contact between your saliva and the gum tissues while sleeping. This helps to protect the gums from contracting infection due to reduced salivary contact. This will also prevent you from swallowing the denture, particularly if it is so small. If your denture is an *Acrylic* denture, you must always leave it in a *denture cup* or a *bowl* of water when not in use. This is to prevent the denture from shrinking. It is advisable to make a spare *partial* denture to avoid social embarrassment that can attend to accidental breakage of the denture. You may buy a denture cup and a denture brush from every good mouth-care clinic or even from an open market.

CARE OF A BABY'S MOUTH

Every baby ought to be breastfed. Breastfeeding serves two purposes for a baby's mouth. First, the nutrient the baby gets from the breast milk confers natural immunity on it, which by extension also protects the baby's mouth from infections it can acquire from the environment. Secondly, breastfeeding provides a form of exercise for the baby's tender mouth. This exercise provides for the proper development of the baby's jaws.

To care for a baby's mouth swab the baby's gum with a cotton wool pellet soaked in a solution of water and a drop of pure glycerin or a pinch of salt. You may also use this same solution to clean the baby's teeth and gums once the teeth appear. During teething period, itching of the gums could be eased with hard objects such as bony rings or rubber teat, etc., which should be hung with a string round the baby's neck to avoid contamination. As soon as a baby can imitate actions, you may now introduce the use of a soft children's toothbrush and a children's toothpaste under supervision. It is advisable never to leave the sugary content of a feeding bottle in a baby's mouth while asleep. This helps to avoid the initiation of rampant tooth decay.

Children who are up to two years may accompany their parents or guardians to the mouth-care clinic each time they visit. This will allay a child's fears about the clinic and mouth caregivers and better inculcate visits to the clinic, as a part of healthy living, into the child very early in life.

EATING RIGHT

The best way to boost your *immunity* and avoid food-related problems of the mouth is to eat good balanced meals always. Immunity refers to the ability of one's body to fight and defeat germs that try to invade our body. A dietician can advice you on the types of food to eat and the quantities of the food your body requires to function optimally or thrive well. Vegetables and fruits should form part of our regular menu. When you eat healthily, you guarantee your mouth's health. The principle of adequate foetal, infant, child and continuous adult nutrition is very essential to the health of the mouth. The formation of a baby's first set of teeth begins at about the sixth (6th) week of the unborn child's life in the womb. Hardening of these teeth commences at about the fourth (4th) month of the baby's life in the womb. When a pregnant woman or a little child lacks the right nutrients in adequate proportion in the body, many problems of the mouth can result. Some of these problems include, but not limited to problems with teeth and bones, tongue, gums, salivary glands, mucous membranes, palate, etc.

Eating right begins in life with proper breastfeeding. The best-practise in child nutrition today demands that children be breast-fed exclusively for the first six months of life, except where it is not proper to do so because of an illness or some abnormalities in the make-up of the baby's mother. At about six (6) months of life, adequate complementary feeding ensues for the child. This form of nutritional care should be sustained in schools through the much talked about *school feeding* and ultimately dietary diversification through adult life. In this way, promotion of good health for the mouth through good nutrition cannot but become a reality.

Preceding exclusive breastfeeding should be adequate mother nutrition and care (pregnant and breastfeeding mothers). We recommend strongly that pregnant women feed well and take medication/supplements prescribed for them by their antenatal caregivers. This will help prevent the spate of low-birth weights we are experiencing in many parts of the world today. Nutritionists and researchers have found out that low-birth weight infants are more likely to come down with certain chronic diseases like diabetes and heart diseases later in life than their normal-weight counterparts are. Over-feeding/nutrition can also lead to excessive weight gain in an infant. There is a clear link between childhood obesity and a number of chronic diseases. For these reasons, whenever you are pregnant and visiting with the antenatal clinic your caregivers try to evaluate the state of your health by carrying out some tests on you, including weighing you regularly.

A lack of some essential nutrients can reflect in the mouth. A good example here is *scurvy*, which results from a lack of Vitamin C. Vitamin C is abundantly present in fruits like grapes, oranges, etc.

As established, earlier, in this chapter, poor health of the mouth can cause deficiencies in nutrients. The types of food you eat can affect the health of your mouth and the health of your mouth can affect the kind of food you eat.

EXERCISE YOUR MOUTH

One of the best and cost-effective ways to exercise your jaws is to chew something. Food chewing can do. Plan your meals to include foods you can chew. Fibrous fruits' used as desserts after major meals can help exercise the jaws. A modern research claims chewing alone can aid *re-mineralization*. Re-mineralization is the re-incorporation of minerals lost by a tooth during the process of tooth decay back into the tooth. This arrests the process of tooth decay! Chewing a sugar-less chewing gum can also help exercise the jaws. Sugar-less chewing gum are readily available in our markets today. Get some to promote your mouth's health.

LIPS CARE

Keep your lips clean, supple and attractive. It is good to apply lubricants to the lips during dry seasons. Dry, flaky and broken lips are aesthetically ugly and damaging to the health of the mouth.

Many lip balms are available in the market. You should select from the range on sale to keep your lips as sweet as you met them!

A simple balm like *rubb balm* or a preparation like the *bonjella* can heal, soften and assuage pain in cracked lips.

WATER INTAKE

The body cannot survive for a very long time without water. The body needs water to perform its functions. Acute shortage of water in the body results in some health conditions and can even lead to death if it the patient is not properly rehydrated. For this reason, everyone is encouraged to drink water liberally. This liberal intake of water enhances health. In some studies, and as advocated by some doctors/researchers, water can even cure certain illnesses or conditions. That is what gave rise to the concept and practice of *water therapy*.

When we are getting dehydrated, among other manifestations, we experience dry mouth, decrease in the flow of saliva, dry/flaky lips and excessive thirst. Considering the fact that reduced salivary flow can predispose one to tooth decay and certain gum diseases, we ought to rehydrate ourselves constantly by drinking a lot of water. This is especially so on sunny days or while we are out at work or on a walk.

REST/MINIMIZE STRESS

Stress affects the body profoundly. Among the many manifestations of stress in the body are those that reflect in the mouth. Good examples are dry mouth and lip blisters. Apart from the pain lip blisters can inflict, the discomfort, and other mouth problems dry mouth can portend, they can make the mouth unsightly. To avoid these problems, rest. The need to rest cannot be overemphasized. The best form of rest is a good sleep. When one is asleep, all the systems of the body are relaxed to work as normally as they ought to – without any undue 'duress'. The body needs a lot of rest to function well. So please, rest, rest, and rest.

CARE OF THE PHYSICALLY CHALLENGED AND THE AGED

We have the physically challenged all around us - the mentally retarded, the blind, the deaf-mute, those without hands, etc. This group of people cannot care for their own oral hygiene by themselves. Household members must assume responsibility for the care of these people.

Automated toothbrushes and other hygiene products are available to use for these people. Assist the physically challenged to the clinic, support them during treatments and encourage them to follow through their treatment/hygiene plan(s).

PERSONAL SAFETY/RISKS REDUCTION

The following few hints can offer some help in keeping one's mouth save from injuries and reducing the risks of some mouth health problems that could arise from our daily activities:

- A visit to hospitals in many parts of the world today will convince you that accidents are on the increase. As we try to move ahead technologically, we also tend to move ahead in injuries arising from accidents – whether it is from domestic violence/accident or road traffic accident or unintentional injuries or wars or sectarian violence. Many have ended up with bruised/broken faces, broken jaws, bitten-off lips, to mention but a few. It is good to avoid accidents and injuries at all cost! Wear protective clothing, goggle, cap/helmet, shoes, hand gloves or any other thing prescribed by relevant authorities when working in, or visiting, an industrial facility, ridding on a motorcycle or a bicycle. Drive or ride motor vehicles/bikes carefully, and within recommended speed limits on certain roads. Seat belts in motor vehicles are for protection. Always strap them around you when using a vehicle equipped with them. Ladies should watch the heels of the shoes they wear. Better floors are clean and dry and built to increase friction between the feet and the floor to avoid tipping over and falling. Beware of wet or slippery floors.

- Physical activity in the form of walking benefits the health of the gum and the supporting structures of the teeth. Most medical authorities recommend a brisk walk of 30 minutes a day for 4 times a week. A part from helping the mouth, this activity promotes the health of the general body.

- Smoking, stress, depression, and alcohol consumption are risk factors for diseases of the gum and the supporting structures of the teeth as well as for heart disease and diabetes. Avoiding them can have significant positive effects on the health of the gum and the supporting structures of the teeth.

- There is a relationship between nutrition and infectious diseases of the mouth. Nutrition significantly influences the immune response and the integrity of the hard and soft tissues of the mouth. Nutritional deficiencies play a role in the incidence and severity of diseases of the gum and the supporting structures of the teeth. Conversely, nutritional supplementation may improve treatment outcomes in diseases of the gum and the supporting structures of the teeth, and may be beneficial in addressing associated systemic diseases. Therefore, it is a good practice to take some nutritional supplements, especially during pregnancy, growing up, convalescence and when stressed.

USE OF DRUGS

It is best to keep drugs away as much as possible. This is because drugs are chemical substances that have the ability to alter a body's system. When we do not take drugs in the right proportion or we take them because of certain desirable effects, which may be injurious to the body on the long run, they can be harmful to the body. Take drugs only when it is the best thing to do or the only way out. Even then, use drugs with caution.

Certain drugs available in the markets today do have some expressions/reactions in the mouth. Some drugs may reduce the flow of saliva in the mouth. Some others can even cause the gums to swell.

It is good to take only over-the-counter drugs (OTC). You can buy OTC drugs from any patent medicine store, some super stores or pharmaceutical stores nearby. It is good to get conversant with information on drugs you use frequently. Most drugs come with leaflets. These leaflets contain vital information about the drug/medicine they describe, including information on dosages, when to take the drug/medicine and possible side effects of a drug/medicine. Study those leaflets very well before you take the corresponding drug/medicine. You can always get additional information on a drug from several websites. You should take that advantage. Some drugs are not, by law, readily available for free purchase arising from self-prescription, except you have a valid prescription from a licensed healthcare provider. These drugs are *prescription drugs*. You have the right to check up on the possible side effects of such drugs with your caregiver or on the internet so you would not be alarmed when you experience those effects.

Never take expired drugs. Always check out the expiry dates of the drugs you buy. Promptly and appropriately, discard all expired drugs in your possession.

ALCOHOL AND TOBACCO USE

Apart from the ugly stains they leave on the lips, teeth, gum, etc., and the bad breath they confer, alcohol and tobacco use is very dangerous to the health of the body. Many liver, kidney, lung, heart and mouth problems are traceable to alcohol and tobacco use. Young promising men and women have died and careers and visions have been abruptly amputated because of alcohol and tobacco use. If you hope to live long or if you do not desire to have a hand in your own death, you may need to consider quitting alcohol and tobacco use.

COMMUNICATION

A wonderful African proverb says '*a problem communicated is half-solved*'. Another one says '*if you hide an ailment, you have hidden the 'medicine man*''. How true! Do not keep your mouth problems to yourself. Tell someone about them. We do not advocate that you share your problem with anyone who cannot suggest a solution to it or who would be indifferent to your plight. Share your problems with the right people. The best place to share your mouth problems, apart from your close informed-persons, is in the mouth-care (dental) clinic.

50 'DO NOTS' IN CARING FOR YOUR MOUTH

1. Do not eat or drink very hot and very cold food/ fluid at the same time. This can facilitate the development of cracks on your teeth.
2. Do not open bottle tops with your teeth. Part(s) of your teeth can chip off or you may even secure cracks on your teeth if they are brittle.
3. Do not use a toothpick unless you can do so without pressing it on your gums. Pressing toothpicks on your gums, especially at the spaces in-between the teeth can create favorable

environments in the gums, in-between the teeth, which can harbour bacteria. The activities of these bacteria can initiate serious gum/teeth problems

4. Do not go to bed without cleaning your teeth. Food particles left in the mouth until morning could be a source of mouth problems because the bacteria in the mouth feed on them and in the process release some weak acid/chemicals that can initiate tooth decay or irritate the gums to initiate gum disease

5. Do not continue to use mouthwash tablets/ solutions endlessly without prescription. Most mouthwash tablets/solutions suppress the growth and viability of certain normal bacteria in the mouth, which are helpful in preventing the upsurge of other problematic microorganisms. Continuous self-administration of these products can eventually kill these helpful bacteria and promote the surge of certain undesirable microorganisms, which can colonize the mouth, causing mouth diseases. A good example of these undesirable microorganisms is *fungi,* causing oral candidiasis.

6. Do not swallow *tetracycline* capsules while pregnant and do not give them to little children under the age of 12 years. This is because growing teeth and bones take up tetracycline and, consequently, stain developing teeth.

7. Do not allow your child to suck his thumb. Thumb sucking encourages the child's teeth to protrude toward the lips.

8. Do not allow your child to rest his jaw on his palm(s). This can cause a malformation or malorientation of the jaws because all the processes of jaw formation and joining of the two halves of the jaws are not complete in early childhood.

9. Do not grind your teeth when there is no food in your mouth; else you will wear away the hardest part of your teeth (the enamel) and come down with 'shocking' sensations (hypersensitivity) on affected parts of your teeth when drinking, eating or even talking.

10. Do not use just any stick you find as a chewing stick. Some sticks may not clean well; others may stain or damage your teeth and, or your gums

11. Do not leave a feeding bottle in your child's mouth while sleeping. This keeps the milk stagnant in the mouth long enough to encourage bacterial action on the milk, which in turn releases a weak acid that in its own right initiates took decay.

12. Do not eat sugary and sticky foods without rinsing or cleaning your teeth. This can encourage tooth decay

13. Do not smoke cigarettes/tobaccos. Apart from its effect on your general health, quality of life

and longevity, smoking causes mouth odour and stain the teeth

14. Do not stay away from the mouth-care clinic. Visit the clinic at least twice a year (6monthly) for check up and preventive cleaning of the teeth

15. Do not drink water that has fluoride in excess of the required quantity in drinking water. It can harm your teeth instead of helping them.

16. Do not leave your little children at home when you visit the mouth-care clinic. Always carry them along so they can get used to caregivers and the mouth-care environment

17. Do not lie to your dental caregivers when they ask for information from you during your visit. The information will help them to give you adequate treatment

18. Do not try to manage dental emergencies that are beyond your limit at home. You can cause more harm than good if you do not know what you are doing!

19. Do not use medicines like 'touch and go' on a painful Tooth. It can destroy gum tissues and the *pulp*. The pulp is the vital, sensitive part of a tooth that carries blood vessels and nerves

20. Do not resort to local preparations that *'flush out worms'* of tooth decay. They do not help. Instead they inflict or promote more problems

21. Do not think a baby is a witch/wizard or has a demon when it comes into the world with a tooth or two. To boost your confidence, visit a mouth-care clinic for advice and counseling

22. Do not use desensitizing pastes like *sensodyne* beyond the prescribed limit without a mouth-health caregiver's review. This can lead to irreversible discolouration of the teeth

23. Do not buy a prophylaxis paste (the toothpaste used by your dental care provider to polish your teeth once or twice a year) to use for daily tooth brushing. It can wear away your tooth/teeth substances.

24. Do not brush your mouth without cleaning your tongue. Scrupulous care of the mouth includes keeping the tongue clean

25. Do not play with any advice you get from the mouth-care clinic. Follow it religiously. It is for your good

26. Do not attempt to remove any hard deposits on your teeth by yourself. You can injure yourself besides the fact that you cannot thoroughly remove them well. There are people trained to do that for you in the mouth-care (dental) clinic

27. Do not use only chewing sticks to clean your teeth daily. They cannot clean well. Use the toothbrush too

28. Do not file or paint your teeth for cosmetic purposes. These practises can lead to serious social and mouth problems afterwards

29. Do not try to create a diastema (open teeth) for yourself where you have none. This practise can lead to teeth problems later on in life. You may even lose one or two of the teeth involved

30. Do not keep your mouth continually open and never allow your child to form that habit. This can initiate certain gum and/or teeth problems

31. Do not use toothpastes that have no fluoride to brush your teeth. Fluoride protects your teeth against decay by fortifying your teeth's enamel against decay

32. Do not use 'dental powders' to brush your teeth. Most dental powders around in our markets contain abrasives that can damage the teeth after a long-term use

33. Do not kiss anyone with an ulcer or ulcers on the lips. You never can tell what initiated the ulcer(s). Some ulcers can help spread the infections they represent

34. Do not hold fuel or any dangerous chemical in your mouth. They can irritate the tissues of the mouth or predispose the mouth to some complex mouth problems. They can, as well, pose serious threats to the body's general health

35. Do not evade appointments with your caregiver. Those appointments are to aid the caregiver to give you the best care for your mouth's case

36. Do not take prescription drugs without your doctor's Knowledge. Some of these drugs can alter your body's functioning (including your mouth's) the way you may not expect. Get a counsel to get you prepared for what to expect, especially for your mouth

37. Do not neglect to assist the handicapped around you or in your household in the care of their mouth

38. Do not keep your mouth problems to yourself. Share your problems with the right people. The best place to share your problems, apart from your informed-persons, is in the mouth-care clinic

39. Do not use tobacco in any form

40. Do not refuse to wear protective devices when working in, or visiting, an industrial facility or riding a motorcycle/bicycle

41. Do not put on very high-heeled shoes while walking briskly on very slippery floors. This is to avoid tipping over, falling and injuring oneself. A fall can break your jaw(s) or teeth or injure your mouth

42. Do not rub herbs on the gums of children

43. Do not sharpen, or bore holes through, the teeth for cosmetic reasons. This practise can lead to

teeth problems later on in life. You may even end up losing one or two of the teeth involved

44. Do not walk briskly on slippery floors - to avoid tipping over and falling. A fall can break your jaw(s) or teeth or injure your mouth.

45. Do not leave your lips dry, flaky and broken. This is aesthetically ugly and damaging to the health of the mouth

46. Do not leave the clinic without receiving instructions on how to keep your mouth healthy when you visit the clinic every six months

47. Do not replace mouth rinsing after meals (with water) or daily hygiene with oral rinses or self-cleansing/fibrous fruits

48. Do not leave your mouth dirty, smelling or ailing. This introduces you as a negligent, careless and an uninformed person. Remember that *'you do not always have a second chance to make the first impression'*!

49. Do not hesitate to take sufficient rest each day or when convenient to do so. This helps to promote the mouth's health

50. Do not share your toothbrush or any other mouth-cleaning material(s) with anyone. Sharing mouth-cleaning materials can spread infection.

3

Help Yourself

Even though we try to maintain good health for our mouth, sometimes some things can go wrong. What do we do when things go wrong? What happens if we cannot access the doctor at the time things go wrong? What happens if we can handle some problems all alone at home? On the other hand, what happens if we are supposed to give a kind of first aid to sufferers before locating the clinic?

DURING THE FIRST YEAR OF one of these authors (VEA) at the dental school or thereabout, he travelled to the village and there he met with his paternal grandma. When she discovered he was in the dental school she started asking him several questions. One of the questions she asked was whether tooth decay was an inheritable disease, because everyone in her family had the malady. He naively answered that people do not necessarily inherit tooth decay but that they do inherit saliva type and that saliva type confers predisposition to certain diseases of the mouth, including the predisposition to tooth decay and the propensity to accumulate deposits and accretions to the teeth with speed. She was satisfied with his reply. VEA thinks his grand mum realized for the first time in her life the reason for her (perceived) assumption. In fact, no one had been able to explain her family's predicament to her the way this author did. '*Thank goodness that my son sent this one to the dental school*', this grandma must have said to herself! If this explanation is true and if people are born with the kind of propensity deciphered above, what do you think? Have you not realized that you need to seek to know certain facts or acquire some skills that could help you cope with the inherent traits you have picked up from your environment or precursor(s), which could affect your mouth and or your quality of life?

Being at the forefront of caring for the mouth for so many years, we have noticed that many mouths are ailing. When we first set out in our careers as people who care for people's mouth – even as students, one reality inundated us:

all is not well with many mouths! We often noticed people's teeth first while we talked with them. In addition, more often than not, we noticed the predictors of the diseases of the mouth in many mouths. Many are even oblivious of the fact that they have problems with their mouth. All over the world, many persons have lost self-esteem, have suffered pain and loss of function, or even, have died because of diseases of the mouth.

Diseases of the mouth have constituted problems for humans from the beginning of history. The earliest recorded reference to disease of the mouth is from an ancient (5000 BC) Sumerian text that describes "tooth worms" as the cause of tooth decay. We have earlier said, in chapter two, that the chewing stick is as old as man is, and we gave the reason we know that. Man may have started using the chewing stick because he saw the problems food debris and dental plaque portended to the mouth, who knows! Nevertheless, imagine a little boy, whose mouth is well cared-for falling from a height and breaking a tooth. If he were your child, what would you do? Alternatively, think about living far away from the nearest mouth-care clinic and waking up in the night with a severe toothache and no one is around to offer any help. Should you just stay there and suffer until you can manage to the clinic or should you be able to do something to assuage the pain and plan to get to a clinic? These scenarios show that even though we try to maintain good health for our mouth, sometimes some things can go wrong. What do we do when things go wrong? What happens if we cannot access the doctor at the time things go wrong? What happens if we can handle some problems all alone at home? On the other hand, what happens if we are supposed to give a kind of first aid to sufferers before locating the clinic? What do we do? Briefly, here, we would like to give a synopsis of symptoms of problems of the mouth, probable problems (where necessary) and what we can do to resolve or attenuate such problems. We wish to whisper this to your ears: *what we are about to teach you can help you keep the doctor away and make informed decisions when you need to see one!* To start with, familiarize yourself with a summarized review of common problems of the mouth that cause, or do not cause, pain and some common causes of infections of the mouth.

Short Notes On Some Common Problems Of The Mouth That Can Cause Pain

Tooth Decay

Tooth decay is holes in the *enamel* and the *dentine*. When we do not take proper care of our mouth, certain bacteria in the mouth, in the course of their own normal activities, convert simple sugars in the mouth into weak acid, which, in turn, removes certain minerals from the enamel and dentine, creating fissures/holes. The enamel is the outermost hard layer of a tooth and the dentine is the yellow layer just beneath the enamel. A shallow cavity may not cause pain so you may not notice it easily, if you have one. When the cavity goes deeper into the deeper layers of the tooth like the dentine or if it enters the pulp, bacteria toxins or foods that are cold, hot, sour, or sweet can irritate the tooth - causing toothache. Most people who visit the clinic do so because of toothache.

Gum Disease

Gum disease refers generally to diseases of the gum tissues and other supporting structures of the teeth. It is toxins secreted by bacteria in plaque that accumulate over time along the gum line that cause gum disease. Early symptoms of gum disease include gum bleeding. When the disease becomes advanced, swelling, pain, bone destruction and other signs may result. Advanced gum disease can cause loss of otherwise healthy teeth and inability to use the tooth/teeth involved.

Tooth Root Sensitivities

The root of a tooth or teeth can become sensitive to cold, hot and sour foods or fluids when the gum protecting them recedes. Gum recession is a mouth health problem in which roots of teeth, because of chronic gum disease or trauma/injury or improper tooth brushing techniques, are exposed. The sensitivities may be so severe that the patient avoids any cold or sour foods.

Cracked Tooth Syndrome

"Cracked Tooth Syndrome" defines toothache caused by a broken or cracked tooth. Biting on the area of tooth breakage or crack can cause severe sharp pains. These fractures are usually due to chewing or biting hard objects such as bones in meat, hard nuts, pens or pencils, etc.

Temporo-Mandibular Joint (TMJ) Syndrome

The TMJ is the point at which the lower jaw joins the skull. Jaw movements are concentrated at this special joint. Diseases of this joint can cause pain, usually in front of one or both ears and limited opening of the mouth. The chief cause of TMJ pains are acute trauma (such as a blow to the face), arthritis, or by some wrong movements of the lower jaw, spasm of muscles around the TMJ.

Impaction & Eruption

Teeth pressing together or growing out, especially at the molar regions of the mouth cause pain. As the molar teeth grow out, the nearby tissues can become swollen and painful.

Some Other Problems Of The Mouth Worth Mentioning, even though some of them may not immediately cause pain, are:

- **Sores or cracks at the corners of the mouth** – due to malnutrition
- **Dental calculus/tartar on or around teeth**
- **Dental plaque** (the thin film of bacteria) **deposits around teeth**
- **Congenital/developmental abnormalities** like cleft palate/lip

- **Malignant lesions/tumours**

Some Common Causes Of Infections Of The Mouth

- Poor hygiene of the mouth
- Trauma or injuries to the mouth
- Teething – growing out or falling off of teeth
- Excessive consumption of refined sugar
- Lowered resistance to infection
- Allergic or toxic reactions to some drugs
- Malnutrition or inadequate intake of certain nutrients

Personal Assessment Of Some Symptoms Of Problems/Emergencies And Suggested Solutions/First Aid

BAD BREATH

A. Finding(s)

- Bad breath with dirty teeth
- or you're wearing denture

What you should do

The mouth odour is due to poor hygiene of the mouth or collection of saliva/food debris under the denture

- you should clean your teeth/denture twice a day as directed in this book and

- visit the clinic for further management of your condition

B. Finding(s)
- Bad breath with
- cold or sore throat/tongue

What you should do
This is a symptom of infection. Do nothing, the bad breath will go away when the infection resolves; but if the condition persists or is getting worse, get medical attention

C. Finding(s)
Breathe that smells like oranges

What you should do
There is much sugar in your blood and this is probably due to diabetes. See your doctor immediately

D. Finding(s)
Breathe that smells like ammonia (choking, pungent smell)

What you should do
Suspect kidney problem. See your doctor immediately

E. Finding(s)
Bad breath after taking a particular food/fluid

What you should do
This is normal as the mouth (naturally) reflects the aroma/odour of food/fluid recently consumed. This breath goes away after a short while with some food/fluid. With some, it does not. Rinse or clean the mouth to eliminate this breath. If it still does not go away, you

may use a mouth deodorant – though this should not become a habit

F. Finding(s)
- Bad breath
- bleeding or toothache when eating hot, cold or sweet foods

What you should do
Your gum should be inflamed

- gargle your mouth with warm water-saline solution after meals and
- visit the mouth-care clinic/centre for immediate management of the condition

G. Finding(s)
- Bad breath
- poor oral hygiene (deposits of dental calculus/ tartar, stains, etc)

What you should do
Visit the mouth-care clinic for routine professional dental cleaning/check-up

H. Finding(s)
Bad breath caused by dry mouth because of use of drugs like some high blood pressure, cancer or angina (chest pain) drugs, antihistamines and diuretics (drugs that causes one to urinate frequently in order to eliminate water from the body)

What you should do

- drink water liberally. You can as well drink fruit juice made from oranges or other fruits, chew a sugar-less chewing gum, or suck on hard candies
- nevertheless, never forget to see your doctor to explain your experience(s) to him

I. Finding(s)
- bad breath
- fever

What you should do
This is a common occurrence with fever or an illness. The bad breath will go away as soon as the fever/illness resolves

J. Finding(s)
- Bad breath with
- persistent cough and bad-smelling sputum

What you should do
This may be a chronic lung infection. See your doctor immediately

K. Finding(s)
- Bad breath
- Fasting or long abstinence from food/fluid

What you should do
This is normal. This breath goes away after you have eaten or had your mouth brushed. If you want it to go away very quickly, you can chew a sugar-less chewing gum

TOOTHACHE

A. Finding(s)

- there is pain in the region of last molar, this pain spreads out
- the tooth is not fully visible
- the gum over the tooth is swollen and touchy and
- the mouth cannot open well

What you should do

- gargle your mouth with warm-water and salt solution after meals three (3) times a day
- take the following drugs:
    - i. antibiotics like Amoxil or ampiclox or lincocin 500mg every 8 hours for 5 days and Metronidazole 200/400mg every 8 hours for 5 days
    - ii. analgesics like paracetamol 1000mg every 8 hours for 3 days or meloxicam 7.5mg daily for 3 days or aceclofenac 100mg every 12 hours for 3 days
    - iii. haematinics like 2 tablets of vitamin C every 8 hours for 1 week
- go to a mouth-care (dental) clinic/centre for further management

B. Finding(s)

There is pain in the space in-between the teeth. The part of the gum in this space is swollen. There is no hole on any tooth and no tooth is shaky but there is a foreign body in the gum

What you should do

- be calm
- if the foreign body is visible and you can remove it, do so
- take a little analgesic like paracetamol or any other one
- gargle your mouth with warm water-saline solution after meals three times a day
- if foreign body is not visible or is absent, go to a clinic

C. Finding(s)

- intermittent pain that is worse when chewing or drinking cold or hot food or fluid
- there is a hole on tooth/teeth but
- tooth/teeth not shaky or broken

What you should do

- be assured that all will be fine
- go to a clinic for a possible filling or further management as the case may be

D. Finding(s)

- pain, which disturbs sleep that is continuous for a couple of days
- the pain continues even after taking drugs
- there is a hole on a tooth in the region of the pain

- this tooth is touchy when tapped gently with a hard object like a metal spoon

<u>What you should do</u>

- take a painkiller like meloxicam or aceclofenac and
- go to the mouth-care clinic immediately

E. Finding(s)

- intermittent pain, which is worse when chewing
- no injury to any part of the mouth
- no tooth is shaky and
- no hole on any tooth

<u>What you should do</u>

- brush your mouth properly last thing before bed and after breakfast and keep your mouth clean always
- buy and use dental floss silk
- take an OTC analgesic and
- go to a clinic

F. Finding(s)

Speaking difficulty due to pain in mouth or tongue

<u>What you should do</u>

There is infection or sores in mouth or on the tongue

- take paracetamol or any other OTC analgesic and
- go to a clinic for help

G. Finding(s)

- toothache when biting food on a tooth you've recently filled

What you should do

If pain has lasted more than one week, go to the clinic where you had the filling or another clinic and complain

H. Finding(s)
- cheek pain that resembles toothache
- nasal condition
- feeling of pressure inside the head

What you should do
- this is, probably, sinusitis. You have to report to a clinic/hospital for management

I. Finding(s)
- toothache, or continual pain that interferes with sleep
- fever or swollen face/gum

What you should do

This is either an advanced case of tooth decay or infection around tooth.
- take:
  i. antibiotics like Lincomycin or Ampiclox (ampicillin and cloxacillin) 500mg every 8 hours for 5 days and Metronidazole 400mg every 8 hours for 5 days
  ii. an analgesic like Diclofenac sodium (or diclofenac potassium for known hypertensives) 100mg daily for 3 days or meloxicam 7.5mg daily for 3 days or aceclofenac 100mg every 12 hours for 3 days

iii. haematinics like 2 tablets of vitamin C every 8 hours for 1 week
- go to the mouth-care clinic

J. Finding(s)
- Tooth or jaw ache as well as
- earache

What you should do
This is due to tooth or gum infection or inflammation of jaw-joint. Go straight to the mouth-care clinic/centre for prompt care

K. Finding(s)
- gnawing pain in the lower teeth and neck
- chest discomfort beneath breastbone
- shoulder/arm pain
- excessive sweating

What you should do
These are signs of insufficient supply of oxygen to the heart. Call your doctor or an ambulance or ask someone to take you to the hospital immediately

BLEEDING GUMS

A. Finding(s)
- your gums bleed and
- you are pregnant

What you should do
- maintain good hygiene of your mouth and
- eat well

B. Finding(s)
- gums bleed
- poor oral hygiene or you have not been to the clinic for more than six (6) months

What you should do
- maintain good hygiene of your mouth
- eat well
- visit the clinic

C. Finding(s)
- gums bleed easily
- you always feel tired
- you have low fever and
- have been confirmed to have insufficient blood (anaemia)

What you should do
This may be cancer (like leukaemia).
- maintain good hygiene of your mouth, eat well, and visit the clinic or any hospital nearby now!

SWELLING

A. Finding(s)
- pale painless lump in the mouth
- lump may enlarge, ulcerate and bleed

What you should do
- this may be cancer of the mouth
- go to a clinic/hospital immediately for evaluation and management

B. Finding(s)
- any swelling at all
- any associated symptoms

What you should do
- run to the clinic immediately

DRY MOUTH

A. Finding(s)
- dry mouth
- use of drugs

What you should do
- If the drugs were not prescribed in a clinic/hospital, stop taking them and visit a health facility to discuss your experience with a health worker
- If you had a valid prescription from a health facility before you bought the drugs, go back to the facility and see the officer, who prescribed them.

B. Finding(s)
- dry mouth
- stress or apprehension

What you should do
- normal occurrence with stress/apprehension
- try to rest/relax

C. Finding(s)
- dry mouth

- decreased urination or sweating
- severe thirst

What you should do

- this is dehydration
- try to rest/relax/minimise stress
- drink water/sugar-salt solution (ORS) liberally
- if you're still not relieved, go to a clinic/ hospital

D. Finding(s)

- dry mouth
- elderly

What you should do

- normal occurrence with age
- try some mouth lubricants in the market
- seek the advice of your caregiver

E. Finding(s)

- dry mouth
- dry eyes
- parotid gland enlargement

What you should do

- this may be Sjögren syndrome
- see a doctor

EXCESSIVE SALIVATION

A. Finding(s)

- excessive salivation
- pregnancy

What you should do

- normal with pregnancy in some women
- try to accept the condition
- eat some dry snacks
- when some women take some nuts or some other things, which are not known to injure them or their babies, they are relieved

B. Finding(s)

- excessive salivation
- foreign body in the mouth

What you should do

- remove the foreign body
- if you must keep the foreign body in place, you will get used to it and the condition will be assuaged

C. Finding(s)

- excessive salivation
- use of drugs

What you should do

- if the drugs were not prescribed in a clinic/ hospital, stop taking them and visit a health facility to discuss your experience with a health worker
- if the drugs were prescribed in a health facility, go back to the facility and see the officer, who prescribed them

EXCESSIVE THIRST

A. Finding(s)
- excessive thirst
- long time since last intake of fluid/water

What you should do
- your body needs water
- go and drink water or any other healthy fluid

B. Finding(s)
- excessive thirst
- stress/illness

What you should do
- reduced body fluid or dehydration. Your body needs water
- drink plenty of water and other fluid

C. Finding(s)
- excessive thirst
- use of drugs

What you should do
- drink water liberally
- if the drugs were not prescribed in a clinic/hospital, stop taking them and visit a health facility to discuss your experience with a health worker
- if the drugs were prescribed in a health facility, go back to the facility and see the officer, who prescribed them to discuss the condition

MOUTH OR LIP BLISTERS/ULCERS

A. Finding(s)
- mouth or lip blisters/ulcers
- red, rough or painful areas

What you should do
- a viral infection
- gargle mouth or clean sores with warm water-saline solution
- take 2 tablets of Vitamin C three times a day for one week

B. Finding(s)
- mouth or lip blisters/ulcers
- creamy-white patches in mouth or on tongue

What you should do
- a fungal infection – thrush/candidiasis
- gargle mouth or clean sores with warm water-saline solution
- take 2 tablets of Vitamin C three times a day for one week
- use nystatin or fluconazole or any other antifungal preparation or as directed by your care-giver

C. Finding(s)
- mouth or lip blisters/ulcers
- fever
- use of drugs

What you should do

- side effect of drugs
- discontinue self-prescribed drugs or see your care-provider for advice on drugs he prescribed

D. Finding(s)

- mouth or lip blisters/ulcers
- red painful gums
- gums bleed easily
- bad breath

What you should do

- gargle mouth with warm water-saline solution in which you have dissolved some capsules of tetracycline after meals (never use tetracycline for a very young child)
- take 2 tablets of Vitamin C three times a day for one week (haematinic)
- take 400mg of metronidazole three times a day for 5 days (antibiotic, amebicide and antiprotozoal)
- take 500mg of ampicillin and cloxacillin (ampiclox) three times a day for 5 days (antibiotic)
- take two tablets of paracetamol 3 times a day for 3 days or one tablet of meloxicam once a day for 3 days if the pain is severe (analgesic)
- go to a mouth-care clinic for further management

E. Finding(s)
- mouth or lip blisters/ulcers
- rough or split corners of the mouth

What you should do
- you either lack some nutrients or you lack sufficient blood
- go to a clinic/hospital immediately

F. Finding(s)
- mouth ulcers
- ulcers form an irregular whitish line in the mouth

What you should do
- this may be an infection called, *lichen planus*
- go to a clinic/hospital immediately

G. Finding(s)
- mouth or lip blisters/ulcers
- use of some form of cosmetics

What you should do
- discontinue use of the cosmetic(s)

SORE TONGUE

A. Finding(s)
- sore tongue
- use of drugs

What you should do
- discontinue use of self-prescribed drugs or consult health worker to discuss possible side effects of prescribed drugs

B. Finding(s)

- sore tongue
- use of dentures or presence of an irregular tooth
- discomfort confined to irregular tooth or denture side

What you should do

- report to a mouth-care clinic

C. Finding(s)

- sore tongue
- pain on one side of face

What you should do

- you may have trouble with trigeminal nerve. See a doctor

D. Finding(s)

- small, shallow, painful sores on tongue

What you should do

- many conditions can cause this
- gargle or clean the mouth with warm water-saline solution after meals for one week
- take 2 tablets of Vitamin C, three times a day, 1 tablet of folic acid daily and 1 tablet of Vitamin B complex 3 times a day for 1 week
- -if the condition is not resolved after one week, go to a mouth-care clinic to report

E. Finding(s)

- sore tongue
- hard lump on tongue or in mouth

What you should do

- this may be infection or a tumour. See a doctor

F. Finding(s)

- sore tongue
- diarrhoea with loose, bulky, bad-smelling stool
- retarded growth in children

What you should do

- patient may have poor digestion. See a doctor

G. Finding(s)

- sore tongue/discomfort on whole tongue

What you should do

- anaemia or general tongue inflammation/ infection. See a doctor immediately

H. Finding(s)

- sore tongue
- cracked, fissured, red tongue
- mouth ulcers

What you should do

- probably Vitamin B deficiencies from poor nutrition. Consult a doctor or see a health worker

SORE THROAT

A. Finding(s)

- sore throat
- fever

- swelling on sides of neck toward front
- red, swollen tonsils with speck of pus on surface

What you should do

- go to a clinic/hospital with laboratory facilities for management

B. Finding(s)

- sore throat
- excessive smoking or alcohol consumption or smoke-filled environment

What you should do

- stop smoking or consuming alcohol
- go to a clinic/hospital

C. Finding(s)

- sore throat
- dripping nose
- itching eyes

What you should do

- allergic reaction. Go to a clinic/hospital for management

D. Finding(s)

- sore throat
- hoarseness or voice loss

What you should do

- many conditions can cause this; try and check-up with you health worker before you take any action

E. Finding(s)

- sore throat
- fever
- aches in bones or joints/headache/stuffy or running nose

What you should do

- take Vitamin C
- take paracetamol
- keep nose clean
- if symptoms persist as severely after a week, see a healthcare giver

F. Finding(s)

- sore throat
- fever
- swelling or tenderness between ear and jaw

What you should do

- suspect mumps
- go to a clinic/hospital for prompt and adequate management

G. Finding(s)

- sore throat
- sudden 'barking cough'
- young child

What you should do

- go to a clinic/hospital immediately for management

H. Finding(s)

- sudden sore throat
- redness
- inflammation
- painful swallowing
- fever
- general ill feeling

What you should do

- Go to a clinic/hospital immediately for management

I. Finding(s)

- Sore throat
- Cough
- Chills
- Fever
- Muscle and joint aches
- Skin rash

What you should do

- go to a clinic/hospital immediately for management

WHITE/RED PATCHES/THICKENING

A. Finding(s)

- small white patch in the mouth
- patch feels firm/rough and stiff
- patch is sensitive to hot and spicy foods

What you should do

- this may be leukoplakia

- go to a clinic/hospital immediately to clear your doubts and get care if indicated

BITTER TONGUE/MOUTH

A. Finding(s)
- bitter tongue/mouth
- pregnancy or illness

What you should do
- will resolve when condition resolves
- clean mouth and tongue with toothbrush and toothpaste
- some persons in Africa claim they benefit from using chewing sticks prepared from fresh *'bitter leaf'* or *nim* plant

SHOCKING SENSATIONS

A. Finding(s)
- 'shocking' sensations on tooth/teeth
- worn out or cracked tooth/teeth

What you should do
The name of this condition is *dentinal hypersensitivity*.
- buy a desensitizing agent like the *sensodyne* paste or *denquel* paste and apply it to the affected area before sleep, after cleaning your mouth with it last thing at night and after breakfast in the morning.
- If symptoms persist after a month, report to the mouth-care clinic

HOLE/CRACK ON A TOOTH

A. Finding(s)
- hole or crack on a tooth or on teeth
- any other associated symptom

What you should do
- report to a mouth-care clinic as soon as possible for prompt treatment, whether the tooth/teeth hurt(s) or not

EXTRA TOOTH/TEETH IN THE MOUTH

A. Finding(s)
- an extra tooth or extra teeth in the mouth

What you should do
- report your finding in a mouth-care clinic

STAINS/HARD SUBSTANCE ON TEETH

A. Finding(s)
- stains/hard substance on/around teeth

What you should do
- do nothing
- walk into a mouth-care clinic and seek professional help now

WHITE/DARK SPOTS ON TEETH

A. Finding(s)
- white/dark spot(s) on tooth/teeth

What you should do
- Do nothing
- Walk into a mouth-care clinic and seek professional help now

FACIAL PAIN

A. Finding(s)
- Burning or stabbing pain on face

What you should do
- get to a clinic/hospital immediately to see a doctor

TOOTH EXFOLIATED THROUGH TRAUMA

A. Finding(s)
- tooth fell off after a fall or trauma/injury

What you should do
- quickly check to see if the tooth is whole (no part of it is cut off). [If any part is cut off, pick it up and report to a mouth-care clinic immediately]
- quickly rinse the (whole) tooth with water if dirty or soiled
- quickly fix tooth back into its socket
- take paracetamol and Vitamin C
- go as fast as possible to a mouth-care clinic

BROKEN LIPS

A. Finding(s)
- Lips broken
- Dry season or an illness or dehydration or malnutrition

What you should do
- keep lips clean
- keep lips supple by applying a lubricant like petroleum jelly or 'wet lips' or any other lip formula available.
- eat well
- take vitamin c tablets or some food supplements
- allow time for healing

MOUTH TINGLING

A. Finding(s)
- mouth tingling
- sneezing
- wheezing
- watery eyes
- difficult breathing

What you should do
This should be an allergic reaction.
- go to a clinic/hospital now

B. Finding(s)
- numbness and tingling around the mouth

- palpitations (feeling one's heart beat very fast or in an irregular way)
- shortness of breath
- emotional fears

What you should do

This is severe anxiety/panic disorder.

- stay in a quiet place to have some rest. after you have rested well, symptoms will resolve
- if symptoms persist, go to a clinic/hospital

*Note: the information in this section of the book is intended to supplement, not substitute for, the expertise and judgment of mouth-care professionals and it does not replace a doctor's or mouth-care professional's advise. If you are in doubt at any time, do not hesitate to consult your caregiver(s).

4

Getting Help

A practise is a place where a professional carries out or puts into practise, his profession. For the dental surgeon or the dental therapist, it is the mouth-care clinic, for the dental technologist, it is the mouth-care laboratory. Governments build mouth-care (dental) centres where one may access all mouth-care services. There also exist many private practises, where one may also access all the services of the mouth-care (dental) team.

SOME PROBLEMS OF THE MOUTH are beyond your limit of care at home. In some other cases, all you need do is to give a kind of first aid as was discussed in the previous chapter and then get as fast as possible to the clinic for professional help. When you get to the clinic the mouth-care provider available sees you and you are either treated as your case dictates and in accordance with the expertise of the provider or referred to an appropriate person for further expertise management/consideration. If there is no dental (mouth-care) clinic in your area, report all cases of mouth problems to your local health post/centre or any available clinic or hospital. They would know what to do. Mouth-care work is teamwork. No one can do it all. There is this story, in folklore, about 3 friends namely, *Nobody, Someone and Everyone*. It happened that there was a job to be done. *Everyone* thought that *Someone* would do it; but *Nobody* did it! That is how teamwork is. Everyone on a team must do his best to carry out his role, which will build up toward the realization of the corporate goal of the group.

The training curricular of many health workers and healthcare professionals in Africa, Asia and around the world are receiving enrichment with courses on the health of the mouth. This development helps them to treat certain degrees of mouth problems comfortably, recognise, and refer complex ones appropriately.

We have various cadres of oral/dental (mouth-care) caregivers with varied scope of operations and dexterities.

THE PROVIDERS OF CARE

Three (3) major distinct professionals make up the dental (mouth-care) team. The providers of care in a typical standard mouth-care set up are dental surgeons, dental therapists/ dental hygienists and dental technologists/technicians/ prosthetists/denturists. These professionals do not replace each other in their duties; rather, they complement each other in their work. Different professional bodies/authorities regulate these different professionals (in training and in practise) in some nations while in some others, a general dental board regulates training and practise of the three dental professionals. So all your care providers are responsible to a higher authority so that they cannot behave any how they want. In addition, they cannot take laws into their hands to do anything that constitutes a detriment to you in the confines of the law. In many advanced countries, lawsuits bordering on mouth-care professional misconduct and/ or negligence are enormous. Even in Africa and Asia, lawsuits are growing at an alarming rate.

The other professions in dentistry worth mentioning here are dental nurses and dental surgery assistants/clinical dental health technicians. There may be some other professions in dentistry not mentioned here. The fact is that many countries may develop certain of these professions to meet local dental needs. It is also noteworthy, that nomenclatures and semantics may differ from country to country or from region to region.

We will now briefly discuss these providers:

1. **dental surgeons**

   These are a group of mouth-care providers who, apart from their normal everyday work of caring for the mouth, perform some minor surgeries. A dental surgeon leads every dental team. Some specialist dental surgeons also perform specialist services like extensive surgeries, intricate teeth conservation, elaborate and complex treatment of the supporting structures of the teeth, etc.

2. **dental therapists/dental hygienists**

   Dental therapy and dental hygiene are two different professions but in some countries of the world, like some in Africa, dental therapists get training to perform the duties of both professions.

   Dental therapists educate patients and people in, and outside, the clinic on matters bordering on health of the mouth, help control diseases of the mouth, perform certain minor surgeries, especially on children, and aid individuals and groups in attaining and maintaining optimum oral health. Dental hygienists acquire skills to prevent diseases of the mouth, enhance teeth appearance and ensure good hygiene of the mouth.

3. **dental technologists/technicians/denturists/ prosthetists**

   Dental technologists/technicians/denturists/ prosthetists receive training to fabricate all forms of artificial teeth and to construct appliances for correcting teeth arrangement. Specialist dental technologists also construct other *prostheses/ implants* such as artificial jaws, eyes, etc.

Dental nurses and/or dental surgery assistants/ clinical dental health technicians assist providers of care in the theatre and clinic respectively, while working.

CHOOSING A CARE PROVIDER

Any of the three providers above can maintain and run a *practise*. A *practise* is a place where a professional carries out or puts into practise, his profession. For the dental surgeon or the dental therapist, it is the mouth-care clinic, for the dental technologist, it is the mouth-care laboratory. Governments build mouth-care (dental) centres where one may access all mouth-care services. There also exist many private practises, where one may also access all the services of the mouth-care (dental) team.

It is best to report all mouth problems to the mouth-care clinic except when you are sure going to a particular practise can deal with the problem you are facing. Appropriate referrals exist in the clinic.

TEN (10) OCCASIONS TO SEE YOUR CARE PROVIDER URGENTLY

1. when you have done all you can and a severe pain persists. Or if a severe pain on your jaw seems to radiates your chest or arm

2. when there is a painful swelling in, or around, your mouth, which is filled with pus

3. when you have a sore in, or around, your mouth that bleeds easily or doesn't heal or get assuaged after a week

4. when you have a swelling/lump or thickening in any part of your mouth or around your jaws

5. when you have a red or white patch in your mouth that doesn't go away after some time

6. when you have a symptom that keep coming back after it has gone

7. when you have a major injury to your mouth or lower face or jaws

8. when you are faced with an emergency related to the mouth

9. when it is your appointed time to visit the clinic (routine appointment or a specially scheduled appointment)

10. when you are faced with a very hard decision to make about your mouth's health

THE MOUTH-CARE (DENTAL) MANAGEMENT PROCESS

What happens when you visit the clinic? What happens is very interesting but if you do not know what happens, it can (sometimes) seem boring and you may become resentful.

In a typical mouth-care clinic/centre, you come in, having a complaint. The nurse, receptionist, or physician assistant asks you to sit in a particular section of the clinic designated as a reception room/hall or patient waiting area after you have paid for and obtained a clinic/hospital card/ folder or a pin.

If the practise is not computerized, the dental nurse/ dental surgery assistant or any other staff in charge of the front office of the clinic arranges the patients' cards/folders in order of first-come-first-served basis. They are, afterwards, distributed to the caregivers or doctors (on duty), whose duty it is to see these patients and either plan a treatment course for them or refer them to specialist caregivers/doctors for further/specialist care.

Patients are usually seen in a *surgery/operatory* or a *consulting room.*

While seeing a caregiver/doctor, he poses several questions to you and examines you thoroughly. Your responses and the caregiver's/doctor's finding(s) are documented in your *case note.* A case note is also your card/folder.

Sometimes, the caregiver/doctor may need to send you to the x-ray room (luckily, some x-rays can be done right on the dental chair) or the laboratory to have some investigation(s) done. If your caregiver is satisfied with your history, examination and investigations, he gives a *diagnosis* of what is wrong with your mouth. A diagnosis is the verdict or conclusion about what is wrong with you. After he gives the diagnosis, he plans a treatment course for you. This treatment course may involve your seeing other specialists for further care or the caregiver may immediately send you to a relevant specialist for forthright care. Prescriptions, treatment regimen and appointments for further treatment(s) or reviews or routine visits are determined before you leave the clinic/hospital.

This process may take a few minutes, a few hours, or even a few days!

The time spent in the clinic during appointments or routine visits to the clinic may be comparatively shorter, though, depending on the condition of a patient's mouth or his case.

This information is to get you prepared for the kind of process you may encounter in a mouth-care clinic.

GETTING THE BEST FROM YOUR MOUTH-CARE PROVIDER

To get the best from your care provider, you must try to be a part of the solution to your problem. Tell your care provider all you know about your problem sincerely but carefully. Answer all the questions he asks you without ambiguity or becoming irritated or embarrassed. Gone are the days when a doctor or care-provider assumes the "know it all" role and the patient just sits there as a passive receiver of care. In the world of freedom evolving on the medical corridors, the receiver of care must participate actively in the process that will ultimately lead to the resolution of his own problem. Your co-operation is very vital to the overall success of the whole management process.

Another area of co-operation is that of complying with your caregiver's instructions or advice or treatment regimen. By the discipline of their training, mouth-health caregivers can load you with a heap of instructions or treatment/review appointments. These are for your good. If you desire to have a better mouth or positive resolution of your mouth problems, you must try your best to adhere strictly to these regimens or prescriptions.

Finally, you must open your mouth, spit out or carry out some little activities when you are asked to, while on the dental chair or in the mouth-care surgery/operatory.

5

The Trouble With Your Caregivers

Doctors are no gods. They are mere mortal humans like every one of us – subject to imperfections and miscalculations

YOU WOULD NOT BELIEVE THIS, but is it true!
Doctors are no gods. They are mere mortal humans like every
one of us – subject to imperfections and miscalculations.

In the course of our long career, we have had the
privilege of working alongside several caregivers trained to
give special professional care to the mouth, whose abilities,
judgments and even dexterities in jobs they ought to be
masters of, we have had cause to question from time to
time while performing some procedures on some patients.
Are you surprised? You should be! We have also hobnobbed
with general medical practitioners and nurses/health
attendants and have observed very closely, with dismay, the
inconsistencies and the ignorant practise of some. We have
worked with dental surgeons who removed a tooth that was
not ailing and left the ailing one – sometimes, at the very
heels of the pleas of the patient who cried out: *'that is not the
tooth. It is the other one over there'*, but who listened? *'Doctors
should know the ailing tooth better'*, they must have thought!
A doctor should know an ailing tooth better than the owner
of the mouth should! Is that not, rather, ridiculous? The
present training of many of our health experts makes them
believe that they know what is wrong with a patient more
than the patient, himself, knows! This attitude must change.
An African proverb says *'it is the person, who wears the shoe
that knows where it hurts most'*. Sometimes, a patient may
have a better understanding of what is wrong with him,
at least, as far as his experience of symptoms may suggest.
If only caregivers would learn to be good listeners in the

consulting room! Sympathetic listenership may help their practise marvellously.

Many healthcare providers around the world are half-baked. One of these authors (VEA) chanced upon a student of Medicine and Surgery taking his final examination in a particular specialty one day, and as he stood before the professor and the consultant examining him, he literally trembled. He did not answer any of the questions his examiners asked correctly. The one that surprised this author the most was when the professor asked him to name the first source of nutritional iron to a newborn baby. A question a good high/secondary school student of biology or health science should be able to answer. He fumbled until the professor told him it was breast milk! He still passed, anyway! Discussing this incident with a colleague (a doctor who was undergoing a year National Service with us at our Teaching Hospital at the time), she did not see anything wrong with the young man's fumbling. She confessed that she did not know much when she graduated too! This author was dazed. As we are writing this chapter, this young doctor is probably out there trying to *perfect his hands* – on some persons (poor ones)! Where are we heading?

Some years ago, this same author talked with some medical students who were almost graduating from the medical school. To his amazement, they did not seem to have a grasp on the basic tenets of pharmacology! Pharmacology is a medical course that teaches the action of drugs. He wonders why people visit the clinic or hospital in the final analysis. Just remove drugs from the hospital and you have just a diagnostic/counseling facility!

From experience and information available to us we know that many medical students around the world offer very little or no courses in biostatistics. To be able to read, understand, interpret and apply research findings correctly and accurately, a good knowledge of statistical methods is essential, but this course is either missing or its content is shallow in many curricular of training of medical/health personnel in many nations of the world. How then do they utilize the large volumes of research materials that researchers churn out into our healthcare world on a daily basis? Little wonder then that many practitioners still hold on to archaic and, sometimes, currently defective knowledge that was imparted into them in the medical/dental/nursing/health school.

There is the need for a general review of our medical curricular. Imagine people spending hours studying some courses some often would never get to use in their practise. Ask any elderly doctor or health personnel you see about certain basic things he studied at school and you may be dazed to discover that he cannot remember them now. Is it not time, we reduced the load of some not so relevant courses in our medical and health schools and incorporate some courses that will ensure the correctness and relevance of what we study to the challenges and changes of the time we live in? If you are at the policy-making level of our society, this is your call. Let us make the necessary changes we need to make in our medical/

health education now. This will help our care providers to serve us better.

You are going to have to bear with your care provider. Much of the problem he faces is not his own making. His problems are a fundamental one. Many factors contribute to this menace. Therefore, like chronic diseases, there is a web of causation! The bulk of the problem lies with the curriculum of training and the politicking of the medical profession. Other causes are issues of policies, selfishness and bad team-playing ideals. The unwillingness of arrogant, but relatively ignorant young graduates to ask questions of colleagues or junior members of the dental team to enhance their practise experience is another cause. One of these authors (VEA) once worked with a certain young graduate who was to reduce and immobilize a fractured jaw. While they prepared for the procedure, he did not know (or he forgot) that operationally, surgeons stretch the type of surgical wires he was to use before they are cut and manipulated into the needed sizes and shapes for use in surgical wiring. When this author promptly informed him about that fact, he got prepared to do so, but he failed to grasp his end of the wire with the instrument he was using in the traditional way, when this author sought to remind him to do so, he arrogantly refused, asserting he was a doctor. A law in Robert Greene's 48 laws of power says '*never win through argument, win through your actions*'. This author kept quiet and protected himself from the inevitable out-lash of the potentially dangerous wire when it swung lose from the instrument. No sooner had he begun than the wires swung lose from the instrument! Thank God, it did not locate his eye in time. With this he calmed down and now (even though silently) complied with the earlier advice and the preparation was down without any further incident. Had he listened! Why did he have to wait to be put to shame before complying? Pride. Ignorant Pride. This hinders the speedy development of your caregivers.

This same author also remembers clearly an incident that shocked him to his marrows several years ago. It was his final year at the dental school and they were right in the midst of a typical final practical exam that tested dexterity and general knowledge in Non-Surgical live procedures in cosmetic, periodontal and prophylactic instrumentation. He was surprised when a classmate walked straight to Surgery 18, where he was working on a patient, and asked to know the right working end of one of the most basic instruments of the procedure! This author remembers that he wondered what the woman had studied in the school for years! That is it. Your caregivers are not *all-knowing*. You went to school, right? You had people at the top of your class, did not you? You also had others at the bottom! All or most of you still graduated, so it is in either Nursing or Medical school or any other health institution. All, or almost all, graduate as professionals! Therefore, you should not expect all your care providers to be as brilliant as you thought. Various regulatory bodies are trying their best to make sure the category of professionals who care for the mouth update their knowledge frequently and stay in touch with relevant technological advancement in the medical world. Even though many professionals are (seemingly) 'resistant' to these changes, many others are availing themselves of the modern opportunity for retraining available today. Help them to help you. Learn all you can about the health of the mouth to take care of minor mouth problems at home and only report to the clinic for your routine check-up/ prophylactic care and when things go very wrong. If you learn all you can from this book, you will be a part of the solution to your mouth problems and you will reduce serious stress for your caregiver. Please help them, this way.

6

Pulling Along

To pull one's body along means to drag the body as if against a heavy load or against a resistance. Many undesirable conditions affect the human body; these conditions may, in turn, affect the mouth or cause varying degrees of problems to the mouth. If your mouth is going to be as functional as it ought to be despite any obvious challenges it may face, you need to learn how to cope in times of these crisis

TO PULL ONE'S BODY ALONG means to drag the body as if against a heavy load or against a resistance. Many undesirable conditions affect the human body; these conditions may, in turn, affect the mouth or cause varying degrees of problems to the mouth. If your mouth is going to be as functional as it ought to be despite any obvious challenges it may face, you need to learn how to cope in times of these *crisis*. Below are a few of the conditions or health problems that could beset the body and, consequently, the mouth, and their (suggested) solution(s):

COMPROMISED IMMUNITY

The immune system is the body's defense against disease germs or agents. This system has to work properly to protect us from these germs, agents, or medical challenges. However, many factors can get the body's immune system compromised. Some of these factors include disease, stress, some treatment regimens, drugs, inadequate nutrition or unbalanced diets, to mention but a few.

When your immunity is low, the body shows it in some spectacular ways, including some manifestations in your mouth. The most common manifestations of a compromised immunity in the mouth are mouth ulcers and symptoms of infections in the mouth. If you suspect that you have a lowered immunity, try to determine the cause with your healthcare provider and manage appropriately.

THE CHALLENGE OF AGEING

Growing old can be very challenging for humans. Scientific evidences tell us that many changes take place in the body as one age. Ageing affects the mouth in addition to other parts of the human body and many seniors do not take proper care of their mouth. This can lead to an increase in the incidence of mouth diseases in the elderly. Interestingly, diseases of the mouth adversely affect the quality of life of individuals. The normal process of aging and diseases of the mouth can cause

- Pain,
- Difficulty in chewing or speaking or swallowing,
- Difficulty in maintaining a balanced diet,
- A distortion of one's appearance.
- Anxiety and depression as a result of altered appearance
- In the mouth, about 2/3rd of the taste buds die by age 70. You can imagine the effect of this on an individual's perception of food palatability.
- Dryness of the mouth due to decreased salivary flow
- loss of teeth and gum tone in mouth with poor hygiene of the mouth, etc.
- The need to wear artificial tooth/teeth
- Wearing away of the enamel of the teeth, making the teeth vulnerable to damage, decay or hypersensitivity

- Diseases of the gum and the supporting structures of the teeth, especially if an individual has poor hygiene of the mouth, smokes or has certain disorders like diabetes mellitus, poor nutrition, cancer of the blood cells or AIDS

To combat all these challenges of aging, you will need to adhere more strictly to the entire message of this book as you age. Read it repeatedly, until you become conversant with its salient points and instructions. Set out to give yourself wholly to the religious performance of every counsel given in this book. Your senior life would be better, sweeter and qualitative if you do.

DIABETES

Diabetes can lower the body's resistance to infection and slow the healing process. Gum diseases are the most common mouth problems associated with diabetes, and, of course, you should know that gum problems if left untreated could lead to severe pain, tooth loss or even loss of some other tissues and supporting structures of the mouth and teeth. Other problems you can have with your mouth include sores in the mouth, fungal infection of the mouth called *thrush*, dry mouth, mouth odour, burning sensations in the mouth, tooth decay and other infections. *If* you have diabetes, you need to prevent diabetes from affecting your mouth adversely by

- keeping your blood-sugar level within a healthy range, as determined by your doctor or daily reading on a good personal *glucometer* (an instrument for measuring blood-sugar). You can get the recommended healthy range from your doctor or health worker,

- taking your medicines, as directed by your doctor/health worker
- maintaining scrupulous hygiene of the mouth as outlined in chapter two,
- stopping cigarette/tobacco use,
- visiting the mouth-care clinic regularly for check-ups and routine mouth cleaning (every six months), while also seeing your doctor/health worker regularly
- eating a healthy diet,

PREGNANCY

Pregnancy poses many challenges to the human body, and consequently, the mouth. Much of the mouth problems that a woman may present with during a pregnancy may be partly due to poor hygiene of the mouth or a surge in hormones levels (like progesterone, which increases about 10 times higher than normal) or her immune system may work differently or injuries to the gums or even viruses' invasion. Taking care of your entire mouth is very important during pregnancy. Many women notice one or more of the following conditions during pregnancy:

- **gum problems** like gum swelling and/or bleeding or growth

- **tooth erosion**, may be due to frequent vomiting in early pregnancy
- **dry mouth**
- **excessive saliva**
- **pregnancy-induced diabetes** can also affect the mouth if not effectively mitigated, but recent research thoughts have concluded that a woman who comes down with pregnancy-induced diabetes mellitus is likely to come down with full-blown diabetes mellitus within 10 years of the initial diagnosis during pregnancy. This calls for carefulness, dietary modification and strict adherence to medical advice, consequent upon the initial diagnosis during pregnancy.

Women who began their pregnancies with healthy mouths will see a reversal of most mouth problems after the first trimester or after their babies are born. But it is essential that she

- maintains good hygiene of her mouth as discussed in chapter 2,
- eat well-balanced, nutritious diets,
- drink a lot of water/fluid and
- visit the mouth-care clinic (after first trimester and before the last half of the third trimester) and her antenatal clinic regularly.

STDS, INCLUDING HIV/AIDS

People with STDs or HIV/AIDS are at a great risk for mouth problems. Many of these problems are because of a weakened immunity or the activity of disease organisms. *Immunity* refers to the body's resistance to infection. Below is a list of some of the most common problems of the mouth with which they may present:

- warts on the mouth
- thrush in the mouth
- fever sores
- hairy leukoplakia
- canker sores
- dry mouth
- increase in the risk of tooth decay
- abnormality with the teeth of an unborn child from an infected woman

All these can make making good use of the mouth painful and difficult. To prevent or deal with these problems,

- make good use of the information we provided in chapters 2 and 3 and
- see your physician and dentist regularly for good advice.

STRESS

Stress is a non-specific natural biological response to demands made on a person. Prolonged or higher levels of stress hormones in the blood stream, among other things, lead to lowered immunity, increases in blood pressure and impairment of mental processes. Stress show up in the mouth in different ways:

- mouth sores
- gum disease
- uncontrolled and unconscious clenching and grinding of teeth (bruxism)
- disorders of the TMJ. *TMJ* is the joint that connects your jaw to your skull

To avoid these problems,

- avoid too much stress and rest well.
- if you already have one or two of these symptoms, try to resolve the problem(s) using the information contained in this book or see your doctor immediately.

SURGERY

After every surgery, one is more likely to get an infection because of the breakage in the skin or mucous membranes. After a tooth extraction or slashing off the gums in certain gum problems or any other type of surgery in the mouth, the case is not different. The person who underwent the operation is prone to infection because there is a compromise of the integrity of the tissues involved. This is one of the reasons why surgeons prescribe *antibiotics* to protect them from infection. This is even more important if an operation involves the removal of the *spleen*. The spleen is an important part of the immune system. Removing the spleen confers a permanent reduction of immunity on the patient – the immunity of the mouth to infections, inclusive!

After surgery,

- Maintain a scrupulous hygiene of your mouth and
- Follow your surgeon's or caregiver's prescriptions and instructions, including taking all prescribed medicines as directed
- Report all strange signs, especially a significant rise in body temperature (say 38°C or higher) or a sudden feeling of ill-health even with a normal temperature to your doctor

RADIOTHERAPY

Radiotherapy is the treatment of diseases such as cancer with certain doses of radiation. Radiotherapy can cause some problems to the tissues of the mouth and teeth. Some of these problems and their suggested solutions include:

- **Swelling of the lining** (coating) **of the mouth** – consult your doctor for the best type of *balm* (cream) to apply or rinse your mouth with warm water-saline solution periodically. If pain is severe, you can take some pain relievers. Avoid hot or cold foods and smoking at this time.
- **Pain** - At the first sign of pain, report to the clinic where you had the irradiation or the nearest mouth-care clinic; prolonging this may lead to greater problems in the future.

- **Dry mouth** - use artificial saliva or carry water bottles for periodic mouth moistening. Initiate meticulous self-administered oral hygiene regimen as we discussed in chapter 2, visit the clinic for regular hygiene therapy sessions, fluoridation and dietary advice. Do not use hard candy to remedy your dry mouth

- **Dental caries** - a regimen of strict oral hygiene, regular fluoride application, carbohydrate restriction and frequent mouth-care clinic follow up are essential

- **Trismus** – trismus refers to the inability to normally open the mouth or flex the jaw-joint (the TMJ). If you have trismus, try to have some oral exercises, as prescribed in the mouth-care clinic. A good one is chewing sugarless chewing gum periodically.

- **Gum infection** – use mouthwashes that contain chlorhexadine to reduce disease-causing germs and ask your doctor for an antibiotic prescription. If convenient for you, use the warm water-saline mouthwash instead of the chlorhexadine-containing mouthwash. Warm water-saline solution is the best mouthwash for this condition.

- **Destruction/infection of the bones of the law jaw** - It is recommended to have all dental treatment prior to radiation or at least within four weeks of completing therapy. It is extremely important not to have soft tissue ulcerations, because the risk of osteoradionecrosis is a life-long threat. Osteoradionecrosis is a condition of non-vital bone at the site of radiation.

- **Abnormalities of growth and development** - crown and root dwarfism, root shortening, incomplete calcification, abnormal curvature of the roots, delayed or arrested eruption, and ankylosis of primary teeth. See your doctor for advice, counseling and, possibly, management.

- **Candidiasis** – visit your doctor for management

- **Gum bleeding** – treat as in gum infection above. If your gums begin to bleed while brushing or flossing, report to the clinic where you had the irradiation or the nearest mouth-care clinic, for an evaluation.

- **Salty tastes** - this should return to normal in two to four months.

- **sensitivity to hot and cold foods** - this should return to normal in two to four months.

- **If you wear dentures** - make sure they fit properly, avoid getting new dentures until all lesions and ulcers heal. Remove dentures from your mouth, clean them and keep them in a denture cup containing clean water, prior to going to bed. Maintain scrupulous oral hygiene, including rinsing your mouth with a mouthwash containing chlorhexidine twice a day. All of the soft tissues in your mouth should be cleaned every day. Ask your mouth caregiver for what to use to increase retention of the denture(s). If candidiasis develops, use antifungals. At first sign of discomfort, see your caregiver to remove and adjust or reline the denture.

CHEMOTHERAPY

Chemotherapy is the use of certain special drugs to treat cancer. These drugs kill cancer cells, but they may also harm normal cells, including cells in the mouth. Chemotherapy can often have a major effect on the immune system and may reduce the body's defenses against infections for many months, both during and after treatment. It is important that you visit the mouth-care clinic before you start treatment and keep all appointments with the clinic thereafter.

The side effects of chemotherapy can hurt and make it hard to eat, talk, and swallow. The most common ones are:

- Painful mouth and gums
- Dry mouth
- Burning, peeling or swelling tongue
- Infection
- Change in taste

To cope with these problems,

- Maintain scrupulous hygiene of your mouth as rigorously as we have spelt out in this book, e.g. by using soft toothbrush, fluoride-containing toothpaste, dental floss silks, mouth-rinsing with warm water-saline solution,

- Keep your mouth moist. e.g. by using saliva substitute, drink a lot of water and if possible, suck ice chips
- Exercise your mouth by using sugarless chewing gum or sugar-free hard candy
- If you use dentures, make sure they fit well
- If your mouth is sore, watch what you eat and drink. Choose foods that are good for you and easy to chew and swallow32
- Take all your drugs religiously and report strange or worsening symptoms to your caregivers
- In children who go for chemotherapy, permanent teeth may be slow to come in and may look different from normal teeth. Teeth may fall out. Take the child to the mouth-care clinic regularly.
- People on chemotherapy are at risk of picking up infections 7-14 days after chemotherapy. If infections occur, treat as we already discussed in *surgery*.

7

Extra:
OUT OF THE MOUTH -
the gift of talking

Many things in life depend on how the mouth is used

YEA, YOUR MOUTH IS CLEAN and sound. In addition, you can use your mouth as liberally as you desire. That is not enough. Nature did not just give you a mouth for eating and drinking or playing alone. One of the best gifts nature has given humanity is the ability to talk. Some sociologists believe it is this ability to communicate effectively that has helped develop the human society better than the animal's. The ability to talk is a gift! Do not use this gift in the wrong way.

In chapter one, we introduced that the mouth is a powerful tool for defense, assault, feeding, recreation, rehabilitation, expression, beauty, etc. So understand that your mouth is 'power-FULL'. There is power in your mouth. Use your mouth right! There are potential abilities in your mouth. Your mouth can either make or mar you. Your mouth can either elevate or demote you. It can build you and it can destroy you. Many things in life depend on how the mouth is used.

A story comes to mind. A woman lay, dying of a terminal illness. Since her life seemed to ebb away with every ticking of the clock, she concluded that there was no more hope of recovery for her; she was at her wit's end, and she was soon be gone and forgotten. So she waited… for death! However, she was a Christian. Late one night she tried to think about what would happen to her daughter when she was gone and to her utter amazement, she realized how traumatized that little girl would be and how severely she may have to suffer to wade through life. Suddenly, she faced the fact that her death was going to spell trouble, catastrophe and untold sorrow to her beloved girl. She resolved she did not need or want to die, but what could she do? She remembered the words of her faith's Scriptures, '*I shall not die, but live, and declare the works of the LORD*' (Psalms 118:17 – KJV). She began to personalise and declare those words. This continued until early the next morning; and to her utter amazement, by morning this woman had total deliverance from the affliction that threatened her life and rescue from the power of the grave. The question, therefore, is 'what delivered her from destruction?' We think she engaged the forces of the principle of positive confession with great faith, even though in this case, she was quoting Words that were specially empowered by the Holy Spirit, which were in her human spirit!   Had it been we were writing a religious literature, we would have loved to quote a little again from the Christians' Scripture that says *Death and life are in the power of the tongue: and they that love it shall eat the fruit thereof.* (Proverbs 18:21 – KJV)

It is necessary that you learn how to use your mouth to attract peace, joy, prosperity, health and longevity to yourself. We will not teach you how to do that. Nevertheless, if it is important to you, you will seek out more literature on the subject to learn more or gain more understanding on the subject matter.

We had our general elections in Nigeria last year. During the political campaigns that led up to it, politicians promised to do all sorts of wonderful things. Among these politicians were some arrogant ones, who boasted and spoke with such zest about their victory that it aroused the ire of the electorate. A particular case comes to mind now. This man was a gubernatorial candidate. He was an incumbent seeking re-election. The argument against him was simple. The general rating of the voting public he governed said he was incompetent, boastful, arrogant and morbidly corrupt. The handwriting on the board was very legible. It was best to bow out at that point, but he persisted. He was going to win at all cost – whether the masses voted him or not. He said many arrogant things – until the people took notice of his words, aside some of his actions that were nauseating to many, and vowed that he was never going to get re-elected. Up until the last moment, he believed he would win or so it appeared. The people willingly and gladly sponsored his main opponent, just to make sure he was not re-elected. True to the people's resolve, he failed out. Sources had it that he even fainted when he got news of his failure. His trouble had some roots in his arrogant words and verbal abuse.

People have committed suicide or lost their lives because of words spoken by themselves or others. People have lost their jobs or valuable contracts because of ill-timed or inappropriate utterances. You need to personally commit to healing/soothing words, and avoid coarse, injurious words that can harm you or another person. We do not believe in just confessing positively, though. We believe in speaking positive, factual words. A student who loiters about, wasting precious reading time on flimsy alternatives like playing games and watching films or just socializing should not think he could (positively) confess his way to success. Neither can a woman who refuses to put in her best into her relationship think that she can confess her way into a great marriage. You have to do your best and be optimistic about the outcome and life, generally.

A girl once talked a man into slapping her so strongly on the face that she ended up with a broken jaw! Had she stopped talking! Imagine the agony she went through to fix that jaw. Imagine the loss of quality of life during the days she was recuperating from the injury. On the other hand, imagine the amount of money she may have committed to restoring health back to her jaw. We save ourselves much pain when we talk cautiously. We tell a particular popular story often around our part of the world. A woman kept having brawls with her husband; and the woman always ended up with physical abuse. She desperately wanted to end the incessant beatings she received from her husband so she decided to visit a herbalist (herbalist in this sense is an African *medicine man*, believed to have contact with the spirit world and who can proffer solution to many human problems). At the herbalist's, she was given a little stone, which she was instructed to hold in her mouth whenever she sensed tension was trying to ensue between her and her spouse. Further instruction was that she was never to open her mouth during the hullabaloo so the stone would not fall out of her mouth, as that was to attract serious repercussions from the *gods*. This woman adhered strictly to the *herbalist's* instructions and she was no longer beaten! In gratitude to the herbalist, she went back to show her appreciation to the man for the job well done and to extol the potency of his *charm*, but the herbalist gave her an unexpected response. The herbalist bluntly told her that what he gave to her was an ordinary stone after all! The woman was flabbergasted. What did he mean? Could he be kidding? Why did it work? The herbalist carefully explained that he knew that her choice of words and unguarded utterances must have caused the beatings she received from her husband so he devised a way to keep her from talking during a misunderstanding so she would not provoke her husband into beating her. Consequently, the beating stopped. What wisdom! Sometimes, silence can be golden.

Next time you want to talk, choose your words carefully, except you are ready to face the consequences of using your mouth wrongly.

8

Share Your Knowledge!

*Share your knowledge with those who
appreciate and welcome it*

WE ARE SURE THAT YOU have learnt a great deal from reading this book. If others know all you have learnt, they will be as happy as you are right now. You may have come across some things you never knew before in this little book. You, also, may have seen other facts you were unconsciously endorsing, previously, which may have become actionable truths to you, just now, because you have read them from professionals in the field of mouth-care.

Others need to know all you have come to know about the mouth. Moreover, you could be the person to make them know these things so your knowledge may be fruitful and beneficial to others.

Growing up as a little boy, one of these authors' Mum (VEA's) taught him a vital lesson, which has helped him to date. This author enjoyed socializing. Therefore, he had the habit of engaging people around him in topical discussions, sometimes, oblivious of the fact that some of his company were not interested in some information he had to share. His Mum observed this and counselled that he tried to discern his company's interest in whatever he said so he would not just keep talking to persons who were not interested in his subject of discussion. He did not need more than that one advice to make the necessary adjustments. One of the first adjustments he made was to stop talking immediately he noticed that his guests' interest in what he was saying was waning. This way, he discovered that many persons he talked to were not even interested in some of the things he had to share. That counsel worked. When he had to cut a story short, some of the people he talked to did not even realize he had cut short his story!

My experience should inform your use of the information acquired from this book. You should share your knowledge with those who appreciate and welcome it.

There are three (3) simple ways you can effectively share the knowledge you have garnered from this book.

1. Number one, you could give out your copy of 'Your Mouth' to someone to read.
2. Number two, you could request for extra copies of 'Your Mouth' to give out to others as gifts and
3. You could ask others to request copies of 'your Mouth' for themselves

You could also help us to serve you better. What would you like to see in the next edition of 'Your Mouth'? We will appreciate your comments and contributions to enrich future edition(s).

OUR CONTACTS
BL Media & ICT Services
PO Box 60,
Anyigba272002,
Kogi State – Nigeria.
veadamu@yahoo.com
+234 805 450 2005,
+234 816 321 0770,
+234 812 687 3566

You could also make enquiries or buy copies of this book from:

WestBow Press

A Division of Thomas Nelson

1663 Liberty Drive

Bloomington, IN 47403

U. S. A.

www.westbowpress.com

E-mail: customerservice@westbowpress.com

Phone: (866) 928-1240

Fax: (812) 355-1561

Alternatively, you may order your copies online at

1. www.amazon.com
2. www.barnesandnoble.com
3. other numerous websites you can search out, using popular internet search engines, like www.google.com, www.mamma.com, www. ask.com, www.yahoo.com, etc.

Join a community of health consumers around the world to contribute to, and learn more about, the health of the mouth at this blog site: www.veadamu.wordpress.com